Tomorrow's Cancer Cures TODAY

25 secret therapies from around the world

by

Allan Spreen, M.D.

Roni Enten, M.Sc., health researcher

Health Sciences Institute

Baltimore, Maryland

Tomorrow's Cancer Cures
TODAY
25 secret therapies from around the world

by
Allan Spreen, M.D.
Roni Enten, M.Sc., health researcher

Published by Health Sciences Institute

ISBN 978-1-891434-41-9

Printed in the United States of America

Cover design by Nicole Mellott
Book design by Gerrit Wessendorf

Health Sciences Institute
702 Cathedral Street
Baltimore, Maryland 21201
www.HSIonline.com

Tomorrow's Cancer Cures TODAY

25 secret therapies from around the world

by
Allan Spreen, M.D.
Roni Enten, M.Sc., health researcher

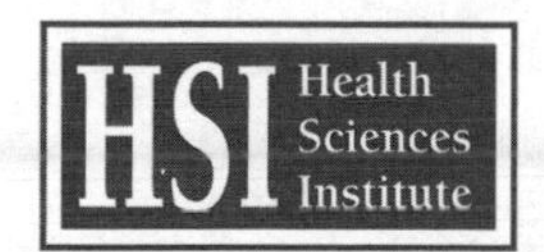

Health Sciences Institute
Baltimore, Maryland

DISCLAIMER

All material in this publication is provided for information only and may not be construed as medical advice or instruction. No action should be taken based solely on the contents of this publication. Readers should consult appropriate health professionals on any matter relating to their health and well-being.

The information and opinions provided in this book are believed to be accurate and sound, based on the best judgment available to the author, but readers who fail to consult with appropriate health authorities assume the risk of any injuries. The publisher is not responsible for errors or omissions.

THE INFORMATION PRESENTED HERE HAS NOT BEEN EVALUATED BY THE U.S. FOOD & DRUG ADMINISTRATION. THIS PRODUCT IS NOT INTENDED TO DIAGNOSE, TREAT, CURE, OR PREVENT ANY DISEASE.

TABLE OF CONTENTS

Dear Friends,

As a medical doctor and true believer in our freedom to choose our individual methods of treatment and healing, there is no question in my mind that we're in desperate need today of viable alternatives to modern medicine's cancer treatments. The rates of cancer are rising across the globe at a frightening rate, and contrary to what we're told in the popular press, *we are NOT winning the war on cancer.* More and more people are getting diagnosed with cancer every day across the world, and here in the United States we don't even rank in the top 40 countries when it comes to health and longevity. The long-standing, conventional anti-cancer methods (aka: cut, poison and burn) that are still being used are "holding actions" at best, and signify the failure of orthodox medicine to really address our health needs and heal cancer.

Cancer Cures from around the World is my response to this need for alternatives, a collection of what I've found to be the best and most cutting edge cancer cures from around the world.

For some of you, the book's title may stir up some skepticism, since we've been told over and over again that there's no cure for this terrible disease. But just because mainstream medicine hasn't found one yet doesn't mean it doesn't exist. My research has shown that that there *are* dozens of cures for cancer out there—true cures—and very rarely are conventional therapies such as chemo or radiation involved.

In fact, my very first experience with the power of alternative cancer therapies occurred very early on in my nutritional practice. One day, a very upset gentleman brought his limping son into my office, an early teen with a huge, firm growth in his knee that had been diagnosed a bone sarcoma. His prognosis was so bad that his only conventional option was a treatment that the doctors admitted was *experimental!* The family had been told that if they wanted to try this therapy, the needed to do it soon, because if it didn't work, the only way to save the boy's life would be to amputate his leg. They were understandably scared and had come to see me ask my opinion of a Canadian herbal cancer treatment they'd heard about. To be honest, at the time, it was far over my head for such a case, and I told him so.

A few years later, a kid I didn't recognize sauntered into my office. He was tall, appeared healthy, and was walking normally. His father then stuck his head in to remind me who this kid was, and to tell me about the family's success with "the Canadian herbs." I examined the boy's knee and couldn't tell a difference between it and the other knee...

I already believed in nutrition, and in the power of herbs, but *THAT* certainly got my attention!

So, after many years of research and using these time-tested therapies in many of my patients, I've put them all together into one resource.

In this compilation, you'll read about the amazing stories behind many natural cancer cures, along with the most essential research about each one. You'll find everything from a formula made from one of the main ingredients in rocket fuel, to a soup brewed from a common roadside plant, to a skin cancer cure made from eggplant. There are special diets which restore the body to health and kill cancer along the way, and even herbal cancer preventatives used in certain cultures (many of which serve as cures, too). In addition, you'll find my opinions (because I do have a few!) on these treatments and finally, where to find them.

Since your health is your personal business and responsibility, I urge you to always *do your homework* on any treatment you're considering trying, and most importantly, ALWAYS consult with your doctor before undertaking any new therapy, so you can ensure the best possible outcomes.

I wish you a fruitful and successful journey towards optimal health and wellness!

Yours in good health,

Dr. Allan Spreen

CHAPTER 1

Know the Enemy

It's been called the disease of our time, and the "C-word" does seem to be everywhere we look these days. Just turn on your TV and you'll find the media is plastered with celebs and politicians who've just discovered they have it and even we, our closest friends, and our relatives are not immune. Though in 1971, President Nixon had already announced the War on Cancer and promised us a cure by the 1977 bicentennial, in each year since, more Americans have died of cancer than the year before.

In fact, cancer is the leading cause of death worldwide. In 2007, 7.9 million people died of cancer. Statistics show that in the United States alone, 1,500 people die of cancer every day—and one in three people are living with it. The five-year survival rate for all cancers diagnosed between 1996 and 2003 was only 66 percent, and if you're between the ages of 15 and 40, brace yourself: Since 1975, cancer survival rates have not improved at all for your age group. I know that with these numbers, each and every one of us has been affected in a personal way by cancer, whether it's a neighbor, a parent, or ourselves. It's up to us to take a closer look at why—and what we can do about it.[1,2]

Before we look at *why* so many people are dying of cancer, let's be sure we understand some of the basics of the disease.

Understanding Cancer

As you may have guessed, cancer is a topic that's fraught with scientific information. In this first chapter, I've compiled some of the key information you'll need in order to feel comfortable with the subject matter as you begin to read this book. That said, you should feel free to refer back to this material whenever you'd like to refresh your memory.

By definition, cancer is a fundamental failure of the body to regulate its own metabolism and clean up unhealthy, mutated cells.

Cancer is also known as a malignant neoplasm (malignant means bad, and benign means good, or non-cancerous). Interestingly, the very process of cancer—the uncontrolled duplication of cells—is quite natural and much like the process that a fetus undergoes when it is forming in the womb, and similar to when you injure yourself and your body has to heal by rebuilding skin cells or other tissues. In fact, cancer is the name given to a normal metabolic function that has become abnormal when it is no longer controlled by the body's immune system.[3]

Nevertheless, we can't expect our body to do its normal cleanup when we burden it with abnormal stress and toxins, can we? Well, we shouldn't, but many of us do anyway, and the mutations that most often lead to cancer are the effects of carcinogens, like tobacco smoke, radiation, chemicals, or infectious agents—and as you'll learn, a toxic diet. And when mutated cancer cells start duplicating wildly, they can ultimately affect the healthy functioning of the body and become a serious threat to our lives.

Cancer Staging and Classification

Now that you know how cancer comes about, it's important to know how it's diagnosed. At the time of diagnosis, cancer is typically "staged" by doctors, based on exams and testing. "Staging" describes the severity of an individual's disease based on the development of the original tumor and the extent to which the disease has spread in the body. This also helps the doctor determine which type of treatment to use.

The four stages of cancer are:

Stage 0: Carcinoma in situ (early cancer that is present only in the layer of cells in which it began).

Stage I, II, III: The higher the number, the more extensive the disease (i.e. greater tumor size, and/or spread of the cancer to nearby lymph nodes and/or organs adjacent to the primary tumor).

Stage IV: The cancer has spread to another organ or metastasized[4]

Cancers are also classified by the type of the tumor. Examples of general categories include:

Carcinoma: Malignant tumors derived from surface (epithelial) cells. The most common cancers fall into this group, including breast, prostate, lung, and colon cancer.

Sarcoma: Malignant tumors derived from connective tissue cells.

Lymphoma and leukemia: Malignancies derived from blood-forming cells[4]

Conventional Treatment Options: A Lethal Triad

Though the American Cancer Society claims that cancer

patients are now surviving longer thanks to conventional therapy, the truth is that people are not living longer after they get cancer—they're living longer after they're *diagnosed* with cancer.

With modern diagnostic techniques, it's possible to identify cancer at an earlier stage than before. Once diagnosed, cancer patients begin a treatment course that typically involves a combination of surgery, chemotherapy, and radiation. Research has shown that, unfortunately, in most cases, this lethal triad often makes a patient sicker rather than better.[5]

Questioning Chemotherapy

Though it's known as "modern medicine," the first member of the lethal triad, chemotherapy (chemo, for short) is really the use of chemical agents to stop cancer cells from growing, with the hope of killing a person's cancer before killing the patient himself. Chemo drugs are designed to kill all of your body's fast-growing cells, whether cancerous or not, and all the cells caught in the act of division are systematically poisoned. I'm sure you're already familiar with the awful side effects of chemo, which include hair loss, violent nausea, vomiting, diarrhea, cramps, impotence, sterility, extreme pain, fatigue, immune-system destruction, *cancer*, and death.

Just one of the disturbing facts about this therapy is that many conventional oncologists (doctors who specialize in treating cancer) give chemotherapy to cancer patients near the end of their lives, even if their type of cancer is known to be unresponsive to the drugs. And, according to a study reported at a recent annual meeting of the American Society of Clinical Oncologists, chemotherapy is much more expensive ($38,308) for treatment of a patient in the final year of life as compared to the $27,567 a patient pays when not in the final year of life.[6] So not only does chemo

NOT do these patients any good, but it actually costs them and their families more than their previous treatments.

Radiation Rationale

It seems unusual that a therapy which causes cancer is also used on a regular basis to treat it, but this is exactly the case with radiation or radiotherapy. The rationale behind radiotherapy is the same as with surgery, with the objective being to remove the tumor by burning it away (rather than cutting it out). But, as with chemo, it is primarily non-cancer cells that are destroyed during radiation. The average tumor is composed of both cancerous and non-cancerous cells, and radiation is actually more destructive to non-cancerous cells than to cancer cells. So it does reduce tumor size, but in the process, it also increases malignancy.[5] And the most frustrating part is that the more malignant the tumor, the more resistant it is to the treatment.

Even if it does destroy cancer cells, the radiation damages the immune system so severely in the process that it's common for the cancer to soon return and spread quickly. What's worse, on average, there's little solid evidence that radiation actually improves the patient's chances for survival.[7]

Second-Guessing Surgery

Finally, we come to the last member of the lethal triad—surgery. In some cases, it seems the most effective way to eliminate a patient's cancer is to simply remove it surgically, but there are several things to consider with this type of treatment, too.

First and foremost, there are always risks involved when you're removing a portion of the body, not to mention the pain of recovery.

Second, in many cases it's not until *after* surgery that metastasis often begins. This happens because surgery disturbs the tumor and causes cells to break away and infect other organ systems. And once the cancer has spread, surgery is generally useless (although it may relieve symptoms caused by a large mass pressing against a nerve or organ).

Remember, cancer is a systemic disease, so cutting is rarely the answer.

The Elusive Cancer Cure: FDA & Big Pharma's Conflict of Interest

In the last 30 years the U.S. has poured $30 billion into finding the "cure" for cancer. Yet, we're still only offered the three options just discussed—cancer treatments with pretty grim outcomes. Did you ever stop to wonder why it is that with all of this money being spent on research, we've been offered very little in terms of answers?[8]

Now consider another fact: A big chunk of Big Pharma's profit comes from these cancer treatments.[8, 9]

It goes without saying, then, that with these kinds of profits Big Pharma won't allow anything to stand in the way of their drug sales—and this is where the FDA (Food and Drug Administration) comes in handy.

Under the guise of protecting American citizens, the FDA (along with a variety of other cancer-related government agencies, which you'll read about throughout this book) can do quite a bit to clamp down on any threats to Big Pharma's profits. For example, the FDA has made the testing and approval process for new cancer treatments so expensive that there's virtually no way any natural product manufacturer can afford to get a natural treatment approved. Tightly monitored clinical trials are essential to

Research Methods 101

In reality, there's lots of research out there on cancer treatments, both alternative and conventional. In every chapter, for every treatment, I've included lots of studies and it's important to be able to understand some of the key terminology in the research world. Here are some key pointers for you:

Randomized Clinical trial (RCT): The gold standard of study designs in medicine, it's considered the most reliable form of scientific evidence in healthcare. RCTs involve the random allocation of different interventions (or treatments) to subjects.

Double-blind: In a double-blind trial, one researcher allocates a series of numbers to various treatments being tested in the study. Then another researcher is told the numbers, but not what they have been allocated to. That researcher then distributes the treatments to the study participants. This way, neither the researcher nor the patients enter into the trial with any pre-conceived notions about which patients should experience particular outcomes.

Placebo-controlled: Refers to a clinical study in which one group of patients receives a placebo.

Cross sectional study: Involves the observation of a subset of the overall population of a larger study.

In vivo: Refers to the test being done in a living subject.

In vitro: Refers to the test being done outside of a living organism, like in a test tube.

determine safety and effectiveness before a medicine hits the market. Today, most of those tests are underwritten by the drug makers. And on top of all that, there's a general disinterest from the pharmaceutical companies in a natural products, which, since they can't be patented, will never bring them the big bucks they're looking for.[10]

It comes as no surprise that the FDA and NCI (National Cancer Institute) claim there is "no scientific evidence" for alternative treatments: There's no budget for proper research and clinical trials for them. You'll see when you begin reading the amazing stories of cancer cures from around the world, that in the very few cases when research was actually done on alternative treatments, the studies were often "mysteriously skewed" to taint results, and consequently the names of these therapies were stained in the eyes of the public. This lack of "scientific evidence" for alternative treatments has also given government agencies the excuse to, in many cases, suppress and harass alternative treatment practitioners.[11]

Stepping Outside the Matrix: Alternative Cancer Treatments

Yes, the truth about the "cancer industry" today is downright shocking, but it's nothing new. Many of the most important advances in history have come from outsiders such as Galileo, Pasteur, Fleming, and others (some of whom you'll be reading about shortly) whose ideas were originally considered to be scandalous by the establishment. Though the value of their theories was realized later, the period between discovery and acceptance is often a long one, and, unfortunately, many people suffer while the medical establishment slowly accepts positive new evidence.

The good news is that there is a growing movement of people out there who have found this suppression of treatments to be unacceptable, and have begun to think outside the box in terms of their own healthcare choices and approaches, so, if you've picked up this book, you're not alone! A recent national study estimated

64 percent of cancer patients to be using alternative therapies and another recent survey at M.D. Anderson Cancer Center, the world's largest with 13,000 patients, found an astounding 83 percent to be using alternatives.[12]

It is in response to this great desire for alternatives to conventional cancer treatments that I have researched and compiled for you what I've found to be the cutting-edge alternative treatments for cancer from around the world. From antineoplastons to mistletoe, from India to Canada, this incredible collection of viable alternatives is proof that the choice of treatment and the power to heal is still in our hands.

CHAPTER 2

The Eggplant Cure from Down Under

Considering the millions of dollars that are poured into cancer research each year, it's hard to imagine a real cure originating from cattle herders in Australia. Yet, 25 years ago, that's exactly how Dr. Bill Cham discovered and developed one of the latest and greatest cures for skin cancer.

The Eggplant Cure or BEC-5, works nearly every time it's used for the two most common forms of skin cancer, basal cell carcinoma (BCC) and squamous cell carcinoma (SCC), without harming normal skin in any way. In fact, 70,000 Australians have already cured their skin cancers with BEC-5, with virtually no side effects—and without any of the disfigurement often caused by surgery.

Cow-Inspired Cancer Cure

It was in the late 1970s in Brisbane, Australia, that Dr. Bill Cham was first introduced to the Devil's Apple plant by a local veterinarian, Merv Gilliver. He explained to Cham that farmers there were using the juices of the fruit of Devil's Apple to treat cancers growing in the eyes of their cattle.[1] Dr. Cham promptly began his research on the Devil's Apple plant, and, eventually, he discovered that it contained cytotoxic (cell-killing) alkaloids with anticancer properties.

Cham later found that these alkaloids also existed in the more familiar eggplant. Before too long, the doctor's extensive skin cancer trials resulted in a formula now known as Curaderm BEC-5.

How It Works

BEC-5 is actually a mixture of molecules that are very similar to human cholesterol. By themselves, these molecules, called solasonine and solamargine, don't have anti-cancer activity because they can't penetrate into cells, cancerous or normal. In order for them to be effective, they need to be able to get inside the cells.

Enter glycosides, a term used to describe molecules with various simple sugars attached to them. One particular glycoside called rhamnose can selectively latch on to receptors present only in the cell membranes of skin cancer and actinic keratosis (a scaly, crusty precursor to skin cancer). As it happens, rhamnose is also found in eggplant. So, when they're combined with rhamnose, the solasonine and solamargine can get into cancer cells where they kill them by destroying their lysosomes (sacks of powerful enzymes that, when ruptured, can eat up any cell from within).

Kicking Away Cancer

The first reported study on BEC-5 compared its effects to a placebo on two different types of skin cancer—basal cell and squamous cell, as well as actinic keratosis. All 28 of the patients using BEC-5 had complete regression of all of their basal cell cancers in

13 weeks or less, while none of the patients in the placebo group had any improvement. In addition, 20 of the subjects with squamous cell cancers using BEC-5 had complete regression of their cancers in 11 weeks or less. And 100 percent of the actinic keratosis group also experienced complete regression, in just a single month—or less.[2]

In another study which used a slightly different version of BEC called BEC-2 on 13 subjects, 83 percent of cancers completely regressed in less than two months.

In 2002, two doctors from the Dermatology Department of the Royal London Hospital who used BEC-5 to treat basal cell carcinoma in some of their patients reported that in both trials they conducted, approximately 78 percent of the subjects experienced complete regression within eight weeks with twice daily use. Only a few patients reported skin irritation and redness.

They concluded that BEC-5 is a safe, effective topical preparation and called it an ideal therapy for outpatient treatment and a cost-effective option for both primary and secondary skin cancer care. And follow-up research on patients who have used BEC-5 shows that once their cancer or actinic keratosis goes away, it doesn't recur.[3]

The Curaderm Clamp-down

While Dr. Cham's Curaderm product used to be available over the counter in Australia, it didn't take long for the dermatologists in Australia to lobby against its use, forcing the government to put it on the prescription-only list (and in Australia, if a product is only available by prescription, it's not allowed to be advertised—so the Australian public didn't even know the stuff existed!).

Recently, though, the product obtained approval from the Health

Department in Vanuatu (in the South Pacific) to be classified as an over-the-counter preparation "for the treatment of non-melanoma skin cancers."

You can find Dr. Cham's product online at www.antiaging-systems.com and treatment consultants are available at (602)490-8030.

According to Dr. Cham, BEC-5 is effective at extremely low-doses and is safe to use very frequently. It's typically applied at least twice daily to the skin and much more frequently—up to 10 times daily—if rapid tumor regression is required.

Remember, though, that even though these study results are very promising, it's important to consult with a physician before trying BEC-5. And since skin cancer (especially squamous cell cancer) can be very dangerous if neglected, its best to consult a dermatologist, too.

5 Things You Should Know About Skin Cancer

Here are five main factors that influence your risk of skin cancer:

1. Skin pigment and ability to tan
2. Heredity
3. Exposure to chemicals
4. Amount of exposure to sunlight
5. Being on an immuno-suppressive drug following an organ transplant

So what can you do to prevent it? Steer clear of too many UV rays and chemicals. Your skin will thank you.

CHAPTER 3 A Fruitful Gift from the Amazon

Originally from the warmest and most tropical parts of South America, graviola has a long history. In fact, if you've been to Central or South America—or even Miami—you may have seen the fruit (also called Guanabana, Annona or Brazilian Cherimoya) sold in local markets or even eaten its fruit. But graviola has many medicinal uses in countries like Brazil, Haiti, Jamaica, Mexico, and Panama where people use it to treat everything from diarrhea and dysentery to asthma and increasing the flow of mother's milk.

From a nutritional perspective, the fruit is high in fructose and contains significant amounts of vitamin C, vitamin B1, and vitamin B2, which everyone could use more of.(1)

But recently Western scientists have discovered that the graviola tree has another big surprise in store—the ability to kill cancer cells and slow the growth of tumors.

I've summed up some of the key information and research available on this incredible tree below, and I think you'll quickly see why graviola is affecting the future of cancer treatment for the better.

Amazing Acetogenins

Western scientists first got their hands on graviola in the 1940s and since then, the tree has been studied in more than 20 in vitro laboratory trials. (Actually, some of the first references to graviola in the United States were made by the National Cancer Institute, or NCI). Most of the research focuses on a set of chemicals called Annonaceous acetogenins, which graviola produces in its leaf, stem, bark, and fruit seeds. Researchers have identified over 40 naturally occurring acetogenins in graviola. And in 1976 the NCI's plant-screening program revealed that graviola leaves and stems are effective in attacking and destroying malignant cells and have a very strong ability to prevent abnormal cellular division—which is what causes cancer.[1,2]

The most recent study conducted at Catholic University in South Korea revealed that two chemicals extracted from graviola seeds showed "selective cytotoxicity comparable with Adriamycin" (a pretty intense chemotherapy drug that's also called doxorubicin) for breast and colon cancer cells. Unlike chemotherapy drugs, which indiscriminately seek and destroy all actively reproducing cells—even normal hair and stomach cells, causing those devastating side effects like hair loss and severe nausea that we so often see with the treatment—graviola has actually been shown to selectively target the enemy cells and leave all healthy and normal cells untouched.[1,3]

Another study, published in the *Journal of Natural Products,* showed that graviola is not only comparable to Adriamycin, but dramatically outperforms it in laboratory tests. The results of the study showed that one of the chemicals found in graviola selectively killed colon cancer cells at "10,000 times the potency of Adriamycin."

Even more promising is the ongoing research at Purdue University (supported by a grant from the National Cancer

Institute) which recently found that leaves from the graviola tree killed cancer cells "among six human-cell lines" and were especially effective against prostate and pancreatic cancer cells. A separate study at Purdue showed that extracts from the graviola leaves are extremely effective in isolating and killing lung cancer cells.[1,4]

Big Pharma Strikes Again

Of course, the NCI and prominent universities aren't the only ones interested in this miraculous cancer-killing plant. One billion-dollar drug company in the United States (that shall remain unnamed) tried for nearly seven years to synthesize two of the tree's most powerful anti-cancerous chemicals, pouring money and resources into testing, and were shocked by the results that graviola really was a cancer-killing dynamo. But this pharmaceutical company ran into a rather big problem: After years of trying to isolate and create man-made duplicates of the two most powerful chemicals, they hit a brick wall and weren't able to. So their testing came to a halt, they shelved the project, and refused to publish their findings in an independent journal.

But one of the drug company's employees couldn't live with that, so that person secretly contacted Raintree Nutrition, a company dedicated to harvesting plants from the Amazon and informing people about their amazing healing properties. Researchers at Raintree went into high gear and began to investigate all the studies that had been published on graviola and quickly made it available to the public.[1,2]

Out of the Forest and Up the Mountain

Recently, an even newer species of graviola called Mountain Graviola has been discovered. It's strikingly similar in appearance to the original species of graviola but its fruit is too sour to be edible. Studies have revealed that although the sweeter graviola delivers potent curative properties, the less-palatable Mountain Graviola has at least 25 novel acetogenins that you won't find in its relative. It also has even more of the acetogenin annonacin, which has been the focus of most of the published studies due to its demonstrated cancer-fighting abilities and lack of toxicity.

Unlike its counterpart, Annona muricata, research on the specific components of Mountain Graviola has only begun to pick up in the last few years. Among the first published pieces was a pair of studies conducted in 2001 and 2002, in which Japanese scientists isolated novel acetogenins from Mountain Graviola to test their cytotoxicity against lung cancer cell lines, in-vitro. The chemotherapy drug Adriamycin was used as a control and results showed that several of these unique compounds (with a specific focus on the acetogenin montanacin) demonstrated potency in tumor growth inhibition that was comparable to the powerful, but very toxic, drug.

Additional compelling evidence has detailed Mountain Graviola's specific cytotoxicity against liver and ovarian cancer, as demonstrated by the string of studies conducted by a research team from Kaohsiung Medical University in Taiwan. One of these trials, done in 2004, tested a range of nine new acetogenins present in Mountain Graviola. Findings demonstrated that the isolated compounds acted selectively against certain human ovarian and liver cancer cell lines.

And in another study conducted by the same research team in 2005, two types of acetogenins were isolated from Mountain Graviola and were tested against eight human cancer cell lines. The compounds demonstrated moderate activity against six of these cancerous cell lines, but the effects were significantly more powerful when the graviola was pitted against ovarian and liver cancer cells lines.[1]

Case History: Daryl's Story

I want to take a step away from all of this heavy science for a minute and tell you about a graviola case history which involved an executive named Daryl at a high-tech company in Texas. Daryl came across Raintree when he began exploring alternative treatments to cure his prostate cancer. A sonogram and biopsy confirmed that Daryl had more than 20 tumors in his prostate. One doctor recommended surgery. But Daryl thought a cure using this common conventional treatment would come at too great a cost. He didn't want to suffer from impotence and incontinence for the rest of his life. Instead, he agreed to a far less invasive round of hormonal therapy (to shrink the size of his prostate) and began a rigorous supplement regimen that centered around graviola.

Within two months, Daryl's PSA level had dropped from 4.1 to 0.00 [Note: For those who don't know, PSA is produced by the normal prostate. Too high a PSA may spell trouble. The probability of cancer increases as PSA increases. A PSA under 4 is usually considered normal. Over 10 is high. Between 4 and 10 a troubling gray area and usually results in having a biopsy done]. A sonogram and several other gamma-ray tests later confirmed that all the malignant tumors inside his prostate had disappeared.[1]

Where to Find It

From a clinical standpoint, graviola still has a long way to go, as its compounds have only been studied in a test tube. Despite the mounting collection of laboratory tests and anecdotal reports about this cancer-fighting dynamo, graviola may always remain an underground therapy. Because it is a natural product, it can't be patented—and without the promise of exclusive sales and high profitability, it will likely never again draw the attention of a major drug company or research lab, so we may never see a double-blind clinical study on it. Nevertheless, there's no doubt that the research and anecdotal accounts that are available about graviola are very exciting, and if you've been diagnosed with cancer, you and your doctor should look at all the available treatment options—including this one.

Graviola is available from Raintree Nutrition by calling (800)780-5902 or by visiting www.rain-tree.com.

Of course, I encourage you, as always, to consult with your doctor before beginning any new therapy, especially when treating cancer.

New Formulation of Rain Forest Herbs Targets Leukemia

As an anti-cancer supplement, graviola has shown incredible promise, but it has failed to show results against one major condition. It is powerless against leukemia.

So Raintree Nutrition has developed Ntense-2—an anti-cancer formula that may help prevent leukemia relapses by stimulating the immune system. Ntense-2 contains some of the same ingredients as the original N-Tense, such as the immune system enhancers mullaca and cat's claw. Both products also contain vassourinha, which inhibits tumor growth. But in place of graviola, Ntense-2 contains three other natural cancer-fighters that show promise in the battle against leukemia.

Simaruba

The National Cancer Institute has known about simaruba's potent anti-amebic activity for 40 years, but it wasn't until 1978 that in vitro (test tube) research showed that it also contains dehydroglaucarubinone, which significantly inhibits the growth of lymphocytic leukemia.[2] Dehydroglaucarubinone is part of a group of phytochemicals called quassinoids. As research continued, scientists discovered additional quassinoids in simaruba that had antileukemic activity.[5] To date, there have been no human studies on this herb, although a few animal studies support the results of the in vitro tests.

Anamu

This plant fights cancer by directly attacking malignant cells.[6] According to Raintree Nutrition, research shows it also enhances the immune system by stimulating natural killer cell activity and increasing the production of interleukin-2, a protein that further enhances immunity. One of the constituents of anamu is coumarin, which may be a concern for those taking blood-thinning drugs. Coumarin can enhance the effects of blood thinning medications and increase the risk of bleeding.

Brazilian peppertree

Also known as mastic tree and Jesuit's balsam, the Brazilian peppertree is a potent antimicrobial agent which works against a wide range of bacteria and viruses.[7] According to Raintree, in vitro tests show it is effective against a specific type of cancer cell that can be found in cancers of the throat, esophagus, and other areas, in addition to exhibiting general anticancer activity.

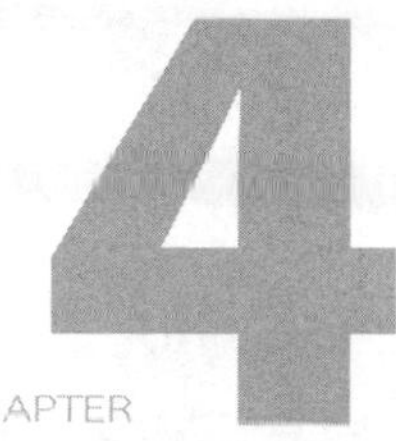

Ancient Anti-Cancer Protection from the Orient: The Chinese Happy Tree

As you may have already guessed, the Chinese Happy Tree can do much more than lift your downtrodden spirits. In fact, it has been used in China and Tibet for centuries to cure everything from colds and psoriasis to diseases of the liver, gallbladder, spleen, and stomach.

Though it's been around for literally ages, western scientists only recently got their hands on this powerhouse of an ancient botanical and discovered that some of its phytochemical components can also precisely target and destroy certain types of cancer cells. In fact, more than one pharmaceutical company has devoted quite a bit of effort to isolating and replicating its active components and, today, the Chinese Happy Tree is available to many cancer patients in pharmaceutical form.

Sounds like a fairy tale, I know, but let's take off our rose-colored glasses for a moment, friends. There's much more to this tree's story than meets the eye.

A Bit of History

The Chinese Happy Tree is native only to China and Tibet, and it's known as Camptotheca acuminata in the scientific community. It's been used since ancient times in traditional Chinese medicine (TCM) for its numerous healing properties.[1]

Camptotheca's anticancer properties were first discovered by Dr. Monroe E. Wall from the USDA in 1958. Shortly thereafter in 1966, Wall and other researchers isolated camptothecin, a cytotoxic alkaloid, from the bark and stems of the tree. They found that camptothecin could inhibit the DNA enzyme topoisomerase I, which appears to stunt the growth of cancerous tumors.[2,3]

Researchers wanted to harness this powerful compound's anti-cancer activity as quickly as possible, and, in the early 70s, a camptothecin analog called camptothecin sodium was tested on gastrointestinal cancer patients in clinical trials. Unfortunately, the patients suffered from such severe side effects that the studies were ultimately discontinued.

Not discouraged by these initial results, researchers continued to work on developing drugs from the Chinese Happy Tree, aiming for fewer side effects. Today, after decades of extensive trials, several relatively safe and effective water-soluble semi-synthetic analogs of Camptothecin have been developed by Big Pharma, including Camptosar by Pharmacia, Hycamtin by GlaxoSmithKline, and CPT11 by Aventis. In fact, worldwide sales of these drugs have collectively reached about $1 billion annually.

Most recently, scientists at the B.C. Cancer Agency in Vancouver, Canada have developed a drug called Irinophore C which has proved "remarkably better in therapeutic effect and less toxic" compared to Camptosar and it's now ready for testing in humans. Unlike Camptosar, the B.C. Cancer Agency scientists say

Irinophore C uses a drug delivery system that doesn't release its load until it gets to the cancer site.

To date, the FDA has approved both Topotecan, used to treat ovarian and small lung cancers as well as Irinotecan, which is used to treat metastatic colorectal cancer, the second leading cause of cancer deaths in the United States.[4]

Take Home Message

Its true that many people have benefited from the isolation of camptothecin from the Chinese Happy Tree as well as the new availability of these medications for the treatment of various types of cancers, but it's important to keep in mind that any time we isolate one of nature's healing chemicals from its whole-plant source and attempt to make a synthetic version, more often than not, we're faced with unwanted side effects. Not only that, but scientists may be missing out on other important compounds in the whole plant source that contribute to its anti-cancer and other healing effects.

In addition, up until recently, the raw material being used to make these medications and drugs came only from the C. acuminata trees, and the intensive harvesting by the pharmaceutical industry has threatened the population of these trees in China. In fact, it's estimated that less than 4,000 Chinese Happy Trees remain in the wild in China![4] So friends, while it's great that the Chinese Happy Tree is available to cancer patients in pharmaceutical form, we've still got a long way to go in terms of maximizing its use in cancer treatment.

Juzen-taiho-to: Another Traditional Chinese Cancer Cure

Juzen-taiho-to is actually an ancient Chinese medicine, and was adopted by Japanese physicians during the Kamakura dynasty (1192-1333 AD). Following extensive clinical experience and pharmacological examination, the Japanese came to regard Juzen-taiho-to as a strengthening tonic for the ill and the elderly. The formulation contains the following 10 herbs, each of which has a long history and strong reputation for its healing properties.

1. Astragalus root (Astragali Radix)—An antiviral agent and general immune enhancer used in traditional Chinese medicine (TCM) to ease night sweats, fatigue, loss of appetite, and diarrhea. Reportedly, it helps counteract the immune-suppressing effects of cancer treatments like chemotherapy. It also helps lower blood pressure, improve circulation, and prevent heart disease.

2. Atractylodes Rhizome (Atractylodis Rhizoma)—A little-known TCM botanical grown mainly in Inner Mongolia, this thistle has been used to treat digestive problems, diarrhea, bloating, fatigue, as well as pain in the joints or extremities.

3. Chuangxiong (Cnidium Rhizome)—A TCM herb used to promote blood circulation and relieve pain.

4. Cinnamon bark (Cinnamomi Cortex)—Used in TCM to treat diarrhea, influenza, and parasitic worms. Cinnamon is currently taken to ease indigestion and stimulate appetite.

5. Dong quai (Angelicae Radix)—In TCM, dong quai is often taken as a menopause supplement (to relieve such conditions as such as hot flashes and vaginal dryness) and as a blood tonic (to regulate blood sugar and pressure, and to prevent blood clots and anemia). Studies have produced conflicting results on its efficacy and have suggested that it may work better in multi-herb formulas.

Juzen-taiho-to: Another Traditional Chinese Cancer Cure...continued

6. Panax ginseng (Ginseng Radix)—Traditionally, ginseng has been used to strengthen digestion, improve lung function, calm the spirit, and increase overall energy. Modern medical research has documented its potential to strengthen immunity against colds, flus and other infections; to stimulate the mind and foster a sense of wellbeing; and to help control diabetes and improve physical endurance.

7. Hoelen (Hoelen)—A botanical that reportedly acts as a diuretic and sedative, and a moderator of high blood sugar.

8. Licorice (Glycyrrhizae Radix)—Licorice has demonstrated abilities to act as an anti-inflammatory, cough suppressant, and anti-viral agent. It appears to increase blood flow in the stomach, possibly preventing ulcers.

Recently, it has also been suggested as a possible treatment for chronic fatigue syndrome (CFS), since it mimics the action of adrenal hormones that are underactive in CFS patients. Licorice, however, contains glycyrrhiza, which can cause fluid retention, increased blood pressure, and loss of potassium.

9. Peony root (Paeoniae Radix)—Considered a blood tonic, it is used to correct imbalances in the blood, including poisoning, anemia, and poor circulation. It is not recommended for people with weakened livers.

10. Rehmannia root (Rehmanniae Radix)—An ancient Oriental botanical used to lower blood pressure and cholesterol, improve blood flow in the brain, and ease weakness. Some reports suggest it might even help avoid premature graying and baldness.

CHAPTER 5

Dr. Budwig's Cancer-Defying Diet

"I have the answer to cancer, but American doctors won't listen. They come here and observe my methods and are impressed. Then they want to make a special deal so they can take it home and make a lot of money. I won't do it, so I'm blackballed in every country"

—Dr. Johanna Budwig

In 1951, German biochemist Dr. Johanna Budwig introduced a diet to the world that has since helped cure the most hopeless cancer patients by providing them with a nutrient-packed combo that fills in deficiencies and recharges nearly-dead metabolisms. Based on a simple formula of omega 3 fatty acids and sulfur-rich protein, the Budwig Diet is a hard-science based protocol that has healed thousands and brought new hope to sick people who thought they had lost theirs.

I admit, the idea of a diet based on flax oil and cottage cheese is less than enticing to most, and certainly seems an amusing addition to a book on cancer treatments from around the world. But the diet developed by Dr. Budwig has helped many people recover from cancer and other chronic diseases. And her success indicates that this dynamic duo actually has the potential to save your life.

Johanna Budwig's Theory

Dr. Johanna Budwig was an expert on fats and oils and was schooled in pharmaceutical science, physics, botany, and biology, as well. In 1952, Dr. Budwig, who, at the time, was the German Central Government's Senior Expert for fats and pharmaceutical drugs, presented her research on the awful effects of commercially processed fats and oils on the cells in our body. While we all know already how fats clog our arteries and lead to heart attacks, what most people don't know is that these same fats are also very dangerous for our overall health.

All cells fire electrically and Dr. Budwig found that these same commercially processed fats and oils can lower the voltage in our cells, resulting in chronic diseases like cancer.

More specifically, Dr Budwig showed that when unsaturated fats have been chemically treated, their unsaturated qualities are destroyed and their field of electrons is removed, destroying the fats' ability to associate with proteins and to dissolve in the water-based fluids of our bodies.

So how does all this this relate to cancer? Well, Dr Budwig also noted that tumors often form in areas of the body which normally host many growth processes, such as in the skin and the GI tract, and the lack of electron- rich, highly unsaturated fats disturbs proper cell growth, ultimately resulting in the formation of tumors.

But Dr. Budwig discovered that a few simple foods can help fix the stagnated growth processes in our cells. She found that when you combine flaxseed oil, with its powerful healing nature of essential electron-rich unsaturated fats, plus cottage cheese, which is rich in sulfur protein, it produces a chemical reaction which makes the oil water soluble and easily absorbed into the cell membranes.[1]

The Facts on Flax

Flaxseeds and flaxseed oil contain substances that promote good health, particularly alpha-linolenic acid (ALA), an essential fatty acid that is beneficial for heart disease, inflammatory bowel disease, arthritis, and a variety of other health conditions. In addition to ALA, flaxseeds also contains a group of chemicals called lignans which appear to play a role in the prevention of cancer.[2]

In fact, researchers have found that a diet supplemented with flaxseed may reduce the formation, growth, or spread of prostate, breast, and skin cancers (melanoma) in mice. Flaxseed was also shown to reduce the formation of precancerous colon polyps in a study of rats. And, in a small study of 15 men, it was found that a low-fat diet along with flaxseed lowered blood prostate specific antigen (PSA) levels and slowed the growth of benign prostate cells, suggesting that it might be useful in reducing risk of prostate cancer.

Another study on 25 men with prostate cancer found that a low-fat diet along with ground flaxseed reduced serum testosterone, slowed the growth rate of cancer cells, and increased the death rate of cancer cells.(3)

Yet another study on the effects of dietary fats on breast cancer growth and metastasis, found that tumor growth was much slower in the flaxseed oil group, compared with mice fed a standard diet.[4]

The Budwig Diet Protocol

Of course, there are a few things you should know before embarking on your own Budwig adventure. First, when buying your flaxseed oil, head for the refrigerated section of your health food store first and try to avoid the high-lignan flaxseed oils (refrigerated, non-high-lignan versions taste better).

Also, as with all cancer diets, you should avoid sugar, animal fats, meats, margarine, butter, salad dressing oils (except extra virgin olive oil and balsamic vinegar or lemon), and all foods high in preservatives, as they are toxic to the body and impede healing.

And one other unusual, but important aspect to the Budwig diet is to avoid leftovers. Foods should be prepared fresh and eaten soon after preparation—within 15 to 20 minutes—to get the health-giving electrons and enzymes.

In general, the cottage cheese, flaxseed oil formula involves mixing 2 tablespoons of cottage cheese with one tablespoon of oil. The daily recommendation is for 6-8 tablespoons of oil, but Dr. Budwig recommends working your way up to the full daily amount. (Those

Get Budwig Benefits Even with Lactose Intolerance

If you are lactose intolerant and want to try the Budwig Diet, consider using the following alternatives to cottage cheese:

- Use raw milk and raw milk products if you can get them
- Use goat's milk instead of cow's milk products
- Use organic kefir
- Take the enzyme Lactase with cottage cheese
- Try Nancy's Cottage Cheese which is made with lactic cultures
- Strain kefir through fine muslin cloth to make kefir quark, which has a cream cheese consistency

with pancreatic cancer may have to work up very slowly, just 1 teaspoon at a time.)

Now, before you worry that you'll have to live on flaxseed and cottage cheese alone, let me put your mind at ease. These are the primary healers, but they're not the only foods you're allowed to eat. Dr. Budwig encourages lots of fresh fruits and vegetables, nuts, and whole grains as well. Extras like cocoa, organic shredded coconut, and cinnamon even make the list.

Patience and Persistence Pay Off

Dr Budwig is careful to point out that her diet takes time to work: It may take up to six months to see results. She also says that even after cancer has resolved itself, it's important to continue taking a maintenance dose of approximately 1 tbsp of the oil per one hundred pounds of body weight, to prevent reoccurrence. And, of course, you should also be sure to check in with your doctor before making any dietary changes.

For more information on Dr. Budwig and her diet, you may want to check out the following books:

- *Flax Oil as a True Aid Against Arthritis, Heart Infarction, Cancer, and Other Diseases*
- *The Oil-Protein Diet Cookbook*
- *Cancer—The Problem and the Solution*

CHAPTER 6

The Acid-Squelching Combo that Helps Your Blood Repel Cancer

Imagine a cancer treatment so powerful it could bring a comatose patient back to consciousness in a matter of days—and needing only $70 per month to get it. This very miracle does exist, and it's been around since the 1930s, when Dr. Hans Nieper began using cesium chloride to treat his patients in Germany. It was Dr. Keith Brewer, though, who took this therapy to the next level by combining it with a chemical called dimethyl sulfoxide, or DMSO.

Cesium is nature's most alkaline metal and when it's combined with DMSO, it directly targets cancer cells, stopping the metastasis of the cancer, shrinking tumor masses within weeks, and stopping the pain of cancer within 24-48 hours.

This amazing protocol is touted by many alternative practitioners as one of the most effective treatments for bone and brain cancers and other fast-growing cancers too. Read on to learn more about this incredible cancer treatment combo...

The Secret's in the Water

Conventional medicine has a lot to learn from the populations of the world that haven't yet been touched by Western civilization about how to maintain vibrant wellness and health. Many of these populations boast very low incidences of cancer, and it so happens that in the environments where they live, there are high levels of strong alkaline minerals in the water supplies. For example, the Hopi Indians' water contains rubidium and potassium and the Hunzas of northern Pakistan have water high in cesium and potassium. It's this high mineral content that keeps their blood alkaline—an internal environment that cancer steers clear of.

Around 1900, this concept of an alkali (low acidic) therapy for treating cancer was developed in the West, and though it worked quite well for cancer, it was forgotten about when only a few practitioners were willing to face the opposition that the medical establishment directed towards them. But one brave German practitioner, Dr. Hans Nieper, believed strongly in the use of strong alkali such as cesium chloride. In fact, in his Hannover, Germany practice, Dr. Nieper used this therapy to treat hundreds of cancer patients, including many celebrities, executives, and even a U.S. President.(1)

Dr. Nieper found that when cesium is taken up by cancer cells, it raises the pH of the cells and kills them. Then, they are eliminated by the body.

Cesium chloride selectively targets cancer by taking advantage of the fact that most types of tumor cells need much more glucose than normal cells. In order to get more glucose into the cancer cells, the sodium-potassium (Na-K) pumps on the cell wall must run 20 times faster than normal, pumping more sodium out and more potassium in. Since cesium acts like potassium, the Na-K pump brings lots of it into the cells. But once cesium is in the cell, it can't get out because it blocks the channels through which potassium leaves. This buildup of cesium then kills the cancerous cell.[2]

The addition of DMSO allows the cesium chloride to target the cancer cells even more effectively since it's what is known as a super-solvent. DMSO also has the ability to penetrate every single cell of the body, and whatever is administered with DMSO tends to bind with it and get carried to the inside of cells along with it—which makes the treatment even more powerful.[3]

How the Cancer Society Dropped the Ball on This Cancer Breakthrough

One of the most important studies on cesium chloride was conducted by Dr. H.E. Sartori, who began his research in April 1981 at Life Sciences Universal Medical Clinics in Rockville, MD. His subjects were 50 patients with widespread metastatic tumor deposits that represented a variety of cancers—including breast, colon, prostate, pancreatic, lung, and liver. Forty-seven of these 50 patients had already completed surgery, radiation, and multiple courses of chemotherapy before trying the cesium.

But after treatment with cesium chloride, approximately 50 percent of the patients survived—including the three patients who were comatose when the therapy was initiated. Pain also disappeared in all patients within one to three days of beginning the cesium therapy. Thirteen patients did pass away within the first two weeks of therapy, however autopsy results in each of these 13 showed a reduction in tumor mass size.[4]

Even the American Cancer Society (ACS) has concluded that "studies conducted in several experimental tumor models in the 1980s found that the use of cesium chloride led to less tumor growth and fewer deaths of certain tumor-bearing mice such as those with sarcoma or breast cancer."[5] Furthermore, they noted that "recent research in rats has shown that DMSO may deserve further study as a drug carrier used to enhance the effectiveness of some chemotherapy agents for the treatment of bladder cancer. Studies done in animals since 1988 have found that adding DMSO to some chemotherapy drugs helped the bladder absorb them better. Research has also shown that DMSO does appear to have some effect in reducing pain, swelling, and inflammation, as well as some other properties that may make it useful in treating certain condition."[3]

What this revelation from the ACS says to me is that (at the VERY least) someone there has most seriously "dropped the ball," as they say. That such a therapy—admittedly effective in animal studies and lacking in serious side effects—would be known to conventional medicine for so many decades, and subsequently ignored, seems to me to smack of some serious negligence (or worse) on someone's part. But, I digress...

The Cesium Chloride & DMSO Protocol

If you decide to try it, the cesium chloride and DMSO combo can be used topically or orally. The protocol can be self-administered, but I *strongly suggest* that you opt to do it under the guidance of an experienced professional.

If using the duo topically, it can be applied to the skin in a localized area (such as the abdomen) using a spray bottle. You should know, though, that DMSO is sulfur-based and has a pungent sulfur smell that is definitely noticeable—and not very pleasant.[3]

Cesium chloride supplements are also available in pill form in a wide range of doses. Keep in mind, though, that cesium chloride along with a high pH diet causes potassium depletion, so it's essential to get plenty of potassium (from food and supplements) while you're on the protocol.

The recommended dosage of Cesium chloride is 1-6 g/day. Most patients take 3 g a day, always with food. Below is one version of a cesium chloride protocol, but as always, DO consult with an experienced practitioner before starting!

Breakfast: Cesium chloride (1 gram), vitamin C (1,000 milligrams), zinc (25 - 30 milligrams), one potassium capsule as prescribed by a physician

Lunch: Vitamin C (1,000 milligrams)

Dinner: Cesium chloride (1 gram), vitamin C (1,000 milligrams)

Before bed, after eating two slices of bread: Cesium chloride (1 gram), vitamin C (1,000 milligrams)

Side Effects & Important Notes

As mentioned above, you'll need to supplement potassium in your diet to increase your blood potassium levels. However, if your serum potassium gets too high, then hyperkalemia (excess potassium) can result, so be sure to have this delicate balance of serum potassium checked every couple of weeks to avoid damage to your kidneys if you choose to try this treatment. Cesium chloride does stay in your body for a couple of months even after you stop taking it, so be sure to continue potassium supplementation for a couple of months after you discontinue cesium therapy.

Since cesium chloride and DMSO cause the death of many cancer cells at once, your body's ability to process and eliminate the byproducts of this massive cellular death may cause a "detoxification reaction" which results in flu like symptoms, headache, nausea, and skin rash. For some people, the herb milk thistle can be very helpful to the liver in the elimination of toxins.[4]

In rare cases, cesium capsules can cause perforation of the stomach or small intestine if the capsules become positioned against the wall of either organ. This is the reason cesium must always be taken with food. Personally, I would use the liquid form of cesium to avoid this problem altogether.

Another condition observed after cesium therapy is a striking rise in blood uric acid levels caused by the release of DNA from all of the dead cancer cells (DNA is metabolized into uric acid). This has the potential to cause decreased kidney function because large amounts of uric acid appearing in kidney tubules can form crystals that block the tubules. This can be prevented by using the pharmaceutical drug Xyloprim (allopurinol) before and with cesium treatment, so that excessively high values of uric acid do not build up.[4]

I must also mention that in a small number of people, cesium chloride has also been linked with ventricular tachycardia, a rapid and irregular heartbeat that can lead to sudden cardiac death.[2]

Also, several physicians that the administration of just .5 g per day of cesium can actually enhance the rate of tumor growth, since this low amount raises a cell's pH into the "high mitosis," or cell division, range. But the data so far reveal that any quantity of 3.0 g or above will be effective for cancer.[2]

And one more important note for brain cancer patients: Brain cancer presents a difficult problem for any cancer treatment, whether orthodox or alternative. When a cancer cell is dying, from whatever cause, it can create inflammation in the brain which can cause a seizure, so it is even more important for you to solicit the care of a knowledgeable practitioner to support you during this treatment.

This seems like a long list of caveats, but if you're interested in trying cesium chloride, getting the help you need may only be a phone call or mouse-click away. Check out the professional support from www.essense of life.com or (800)760 1947.

Cesium Chloride and DMSO can be purchased through the following resource:

- www.shopthewolfeclinic.com

CHAPTER 7

A Nutrition Revolution: Max Gerson's Cancer Detox Diet

Do you remember the famous words of Hippocrates who once advised that we let food be our medicine? Well, there's a growing movement of people out there who have made this piece of ancient wisdom their mantra, taking the age-old advice literally—and reversing their cancer as a result. The wise Hippocrates, also known as the Father of Medicine, was referring to mostly fruits and vegetables as the cure for our ills, and back in 1920s, a German doctor named Max Gerson pioneered a revolutionary diet based on this philosophy that quickly revealed itself to be a potent nutritional and metabolic therapy—*and a cure for cancer.*

For over 60 years, the Gerson therapy has blended a diet of organic fruits and vegetables and fresh juices with special detoxification methods to help thousands of people recover from cancer. Of course, this success came much to the dismay of the FDA and the American Medical Association (AMA), who turned on the heat and harassed Gerson as his discovery became publicized, even threatening to squash his incredible findings.

But against all odds, the Gerson therapy has survived and thrived—

and the diet, along with the great doctor's legacy, live on through Gerson's daughter, Charlotte, and the Gerson clinic in Tijuana, Mexico. The facility serves both as a testament to the therapy's power to heal cancer, and a beacon of hope for patients across the globe.

The Great Gerson

Dr. Max Gerson's fascination with healing diets began with his pursuit of a cure for his own migraines. After years of intensive research, he developed what he found to be the perfect migraine-healing diet. But, soon after, Gerson discovered his diet could also cure skin tuberculosis. He went on to successfully treat numerous skin TB patients, even establishing a special treatment program at the Munich University Hospital, where a clinical trial found that 446 out of 450 skin tuberculosis patients on the Gerson diet recovered completely. Dr. Gerson and Dr. Sauerbruch, a famous surgeon, published their findings in leading medical journals and established the Gerson therapy as the first cure for skin tuberculosis.(1)

Dr. Gerson's success quickly gained the attention of Nobel Prize winner, Albert Schweitzer, M.D., whose wife was cured of lung tuberculosis with the diet therapy after all conventional treatments had failed her. Dr. Schweitzer, whose own Type II diabetes was also cured by the Gerson treatment, later observed the successful application of the dietary therapy to heart disease, kidney failure, and finally—cancer. After Dr. Gerson immigrated to America in the 1930s, he treated hundreds of terminal cancer patients and incredibly, only eight years later, presented his recovered patients before Congress.

The Theory Behind the Therapy

Before moving forward, I want to take a minute to make sure you understand the connection between diet and cancer. When the body can't properly process foods and when defenses are low, we get sick. But what causes our metabolism to go haywire in the first place? Poor nutrition, exposure to chemicals, and cooking methods that destroy nutrients are just a few of the reasons our bodies get bogged down. And Max Gerson believed these reasons, plus a combination of degenerated liver and pancreatic functions, cause the body's immune system to break down, giving cancer a perfect opportunity to flourish. He also believed cancer could be controlled in the presence of a healthy liver and with a proper balance of sodium and potassium in the body.

Gerson hypothesized that a sick body quickly becomes overtaken by sodium—but with the implementation of the Gerson diet, potassium could be built up and sodium could be excreted, thus returning us to our natural balance.

So, the Gerson Diet is a metabolic therapy that includes detoxification and nutritional replacement, and stimulates the proper immune function that naturally dissolves tumors. Nutritional replacement in this case is achieved by following a diet rich in whole, natural, and organic foods like whole grains, vegetables, and fruits—and <u>no</u> foods with additives or preservatives like coffee, white flour, and sugar.

Vitamins, minerals and enzymes are also added to the therapy all serving to help the immune system to properly deal with toxins produced by tumors. Enemas, gallbladder flushes, herbal teas and lots of fresh juices are other powerful ways that detoxification is achieved in Gerson therapy.[2]

When he first developed it, Dr. Gerson's therapy was so far ahead of its time that it was nearly impossible to explain in scientific terms how it could cure both chronic and infectious diseases. Since the Gerson diet is naturally high in vitamins, minerals, enzymes, micro-nutrients, and fluids and extremely low in sodium and fats, it's been theorized that the diet serves to boost your body's immune system to heal itself of disease. Though the philosophy is simple, the actual therapy is a bit more elaborate.[3]

Considered quite an eccentric concept at the time, only a few peer-reviewed journals were receptive to Gerson's idea that diet could affect health, but he continued to publish articles on his therapy along with case histories of patients that had been cured. In fact, Gerson's first publication on the topic of cancer in 1945, was almost *40 years* before the adoption of the current official U.S. National Cancer Institute program on diet, nutrition, and cancer. And in 1958, after 30 years of clinical experimentation, Gerson finally published *A Cancer Therapy: Results of 50 Cases,* which details the theories, treatment, and his results.[4,5]

Clash with the FDA and AMA

Shortly after he arrived in the United States from Germany, Max Gerson found himself on the bad side of Morris Fishbein, the editor of the *Journal of the American Medical Association (JAMA),* after formally stating his anti-tobacco stance (it's no wonder Fishbein was upset, when you consider that Phillip Morris was JAMA's chief source of advertising at the time!)

In addition, Dr. Gerson came forward with his cancer successes to the government and ignored the formal stance of the AMA that there is no connection between cancer and diet.

Not long after he presented the U.S. Senate with his cancer successes, the medical director of New York's Gotham Hospital called his recoveries "miracles" and an independent doctor who reviewed Gerson's records for Congress stated that "relief of severe pain was achieved in about 90 percent of cases." Despite these testimonies in his favor, shortly thereafter, Gerson was openly attacked in writing in JAMA, expelled from the New York medical society, and deprived of all hospital affiliations and even malpractice insurance.[6]

The Gerson Legacy: Recent Research

In the 20 plus years since his death, even more studies on the Gerson therapy have been published, providing continued validation of this incredible breakthrough. In 1990, a study of a diet regimen similar to the Gerson therapy was done in Austria where patients received standard treatment along with the special diet. The authors found that the diet appeared to help patients live longer than usual and have fewer side effects.[5]

More recently, in 1995, a retrospective study set in a Tijuana hospital found five-year survival rates of melanoma patients using the Gerson therapy to be considerably higher than normal.[7] Finally, in 2007, the University of Manchester analyzed six case studies of patients with cancer that followed the Gerson therapy. They found that the regimen had positive physical and psychological effects on the subjects.[9]

Incredibly, in 2001—21 years after Gerson's death—JAMA published an article suggesting that the AMA had staged a "Grand Conspiracy against the Cure of Cancer." The author of the article, William Regelsen, claimed that "inappropriate judgments...resulted in injury to good observations," and went on to defend the results and scientific basis of the Gerson therapy. The government even contracted Dr. Patricia Spain Ward of the University of Chicago to investigate the Gerson therapy, and she came to the conclusion that the therapy was one of the greatest innovations in the history of cancer therapy.

But, again, despite the scientific findings in its favor, the Gerson diet continues to be shunned in this country. Though the Gerson Clinic continues today, under the leadership of Charlotte Gerson in Tijuana, any doctor who chooses to use the therapy in the USA is at risk of losing their license.

You Are What You Eat

So what, you ask, does a typical day look like for someone on the Gerson therapy regimen? Overall, it includes:

- 13 total glasses of fresh, raw carrot/apple and green-leaf juices prepared hourly from fresh, organic fruits and vegetables.
- 3 full vegetarian meals, which typically include salad, cooked vegetables, baked potatoes, vegetable soup, and juice.
- Fresh fruit and fresh fruit dessert is available at all hours for snacking, in addition to the regular diet.[1]

A Typical Day on the Gerson Diet

BREAKFAST:

- 1 glass orange juice
- Large portion oatmeal (without milk)
- Bread

LUNCH & DINNER:

- 1 glass carrot-apple juice
- Raw vegetable salad
- 2 cups Hippocrates soup
- 1 large baked potato

- Cooked vegetables

DESSERT:

- fruit (stewed or raw)

SNACKS:

- 6 additional carrot-apple juices
- 5 green juices
- fruit & vegetables

Extra Supplements and Detoxification

Aside from the diet itself, another very important piece of the Gerson Therapy is detoxification of the tissues and blood, and when you're healing the Gerson way, first and foremost come coffee enemas. It may sound a bit unusual, but patients have long reported that the enemas decrease pain and make for faster healing. Dr. Gerson found that enzymes within the gut wall and liver are stimulated by the enemas, and bile flow is increased as well, enhancing the body's ability to eliminate toxic residues from the environment, drugs, and chemo, as well as tumors and other diseased tissue.

Castor oil packs are also used to stimulate bile flow and enhance the liver's ability to filter blood, and digestive enzymes are taken to enhance absorption of nutrients and assist in the elimination of damaged tissue. When necessary, supplemental potassium, Lugol's solution (a source of iodine), vitamin B12, thyroid hormone, and injectable crude liver extract are also used. Remember: it's always best to attempt any and all of these therapeutic components only under the proper guidance.(1)

It All Boils Down to Good Health

One of the key ingredients in the Gerson diet is Hippocrates Soup. There are several variations, such as the addition of more garlic or herbs, so feel free to experiment to your liking. Just bear in mind that this is a great detox idea, and not by itself any treatment for cancer.

Step 1:

Chop, but do not peel, the following vegetables:

1 medium celery knob
1 1/2 lbs tomatoes
1 medium parsley root
2 medium onions
garlic as desired
1 lb potatoes
2 small leeks
parsley

Place all vegetables into a large pot. Cover with purified, distilled water. Simmer slowly for 2-3 hours. Toss out the vegetables and keep broth. This makes about 4 quarts of soup stock.

Step 2:

Strain 1 quart of stock, then add the following fresh, chopped vegetables:

1 cup leeks
1/2 cup onion
1/2 cup tomatoes
2 cups potatoes
2 cup parsley root
1 cup carrots
1 cup celery root (or celery stalks)

Add vegetables to the stock, simmer slowly, until the potatoes are soft. Can be served as-is or after being ground through a food mill or pureed in a blender.

The Gerson Diet Moves into the 21st Century with the Raw Food Movement

Though it's still not entirely clear how the therapy works, one thing is pretty certain, friends: a diet filled with lots of fresh and organic fruits and vegetables is clearly the way to go for optimum health, whether or not you're battling cancer. And part of the legacy of Max Gerson, plus all of the emerging clinical evidence before us, makes for a hot trend in healthy and healing diets called Raw Foodism or the Raw Food Movement.

A raw food diet, by definition, includes food that is eaten raw, or uncooked as it's believed that essential nutrients are destroyed when certain foods are cooked. But if they're consumed in their original form, they will retain all of their original nutrients. In such foods, the enzymes are still fully functional and provide a wider range of health benefits.[10]

Many raw foodists keep their diets diverse with nifty kitchen tools like a blender or food processor and a dehydrator to "bake" breads and snacks at low temperatures to ensure the viability of the enzymes is maintained. Reports of increased energy and vitality, weight loss and clearer skin on a raw or mostly raw diet, are common, not to mention more profound health benefits.

If you do want to make the switch, just remember: raw takes some getting used to and it's best to start by adding one raw meal a day and progressing slowly until you reach your goal (often about 70 to 90 percent raw). Also, be sure to plan your meals carefully to ensure a well-balanced diet.

True to its name, Raw Foodism is an "ism" for a reason—because it's truly a way of life. And like anything worthwhile, healing takes time and commitment. When you approach it in this way, rest assured you'll reap the best rewards.

Where to Find the Gerson Therapy

While many patients have made full recoveries practicing the Gerson Therapy on their own, for best results, it's best to start treatment at a Gerson Institute licensed treatment center. To contact the Gerson Institute in Mexico from within the U.S. call 1-888-4GERSON, outside the U.S. please phone (619)685-5353.

Raw Lettuce Wraps

INGREDIENTS:

2 very ripe avocados
3 tomatoes, diced
1/2 jalapeno pepper, diced
2 tbsp yellow onion, diced
3 cloves fresh garlic, minced
1/4 cup fresh cilantro, chopped
kernels from one ear raw organic corn
2 tsp fresh lime juice
6-8 large romaine lettuce leaves

- In a medium sized bowl, mash the avocado.
- Add remaining ingredients and stir until well mixed.
- Spread 2-3 tablespoons of this mixture onto lettuce leaves and wrap. Enjoy![11]

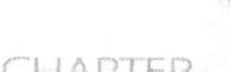

8 More than Just a Christmas Kiss: Wiping Out Cancer with Mistletoe

Ok, I know what you're thinking: "Mistletoe? Yeah right!" But the truth is that this familiar plant has a lot more to it than just the amorous yuletide ritual. Recently popularized by actress Suzanne Somers who used the herb instead of chemotherapy to treat her breast cancer, mistletoe, known to the ancients as "all heal," has long been used by herbalists to treat a variety of health problems, including headaches, lung disease, internal bleeding, nervous conditions—and even cancerous tumors.

In fact, mistletoe is available commercially in Europe as we speak, under a variety of names, to kill cancers of the colon, stomach, breast, and lung. In European countries Mistletoe is often preferred over conventional treatments because of its ability to help repair DNA damage caused by cancer, and to prevent the spread of cancer. Many cancer patients worldwide—and particularly in Germany—even use it together with radiation, chemotherapy or surgery.

Herbal Immortality

Mistletoe has long appeared in the folklore of the Ancient Greeks and Druids as a "cure-all" and may have been used in the solstice-related rites in Druidic Britain as a symbol of immortality. Early in the 20th century, naturalist Rudolf Steiner developed the first extracts of mistletoe for injection. He theorized that it might help treat cancer because, like cancer, mistletoe is a parasitic growth that eventually kills its host. Steiner's instinct proved to be right on: Over the years, about 1,000 in vitro studies have shown that mistletoe or its main constituents do have some significant anticancer activity.(1)

According to these studies, mistletoe has the ability to kill various types of cancer cells while simultaneously stimulating the immune system, thus fighting progression of the disease.

There are actually more than eight decades of research to support the use of mistletoe as a cancer treatment. In the 1970s, doctors found that 547 breast cancer patients using mistletoe after tumor removal had significantly increased survival rates when compared with patients receiving only conventional treatment.

Other studies involving many other types of cancers show that mistletoe is at least as effective as mainstream "cures," but without any known side effects, unlike radiation and chemotherapy.

Most recently, the Institute for Preventive Medicine in Germany published the results of a study involving more than 1,668 cancer patients treated with mistletoe. Patients taking the herb had up to a 56 percent higher survival rate than the control group. Probably the most interesting part of this study was the variety of cancers affected, which included colorectal, stomach, breast, and lung.(3) And a 2003 review on mistletoe identified 23 studies testing its efficacy, and 12 of the 23 showed one or more statistically significant, positive results, while another seven studies showed at least one positive trend—pretty incredible stats.[4]

Making Mistletoe Your Cancer Weapon of Choice

But treatment with mistletoe isn't quite as simple as some other herbal treatments. Unfortunately, you can't simply brew up a cup of mistletoe tea to enjoy by the holiday fire. Although mistletoe is available in the U.S. in herb form, it's important not to self-treat with it, as the fruit of many varieties of mistletoe are actually poisonous if ingested. Besides, the most effective mistletoe therapies are usually given by injection into the muscle (intramuscular, or IM), beneath the skin (subcutaneous, or Sub-Q), or into a vein (intravenous, or IV). In most reported studies, injections under the skin were given 2 to 3 times a week for various lengths of time.[2] And it's important to be aware that injectable forms of mistletoe are currently illegal in the U.S. (they are pending FDA approval). However, as I mentioned at the beginning of this chapter, European doctors have been using it to treat cancer for some time now.[5]

In Europe, mistletoe is marketed under various brand names, including Iscador, Eurixor, Helixor, Isorel, Iscucin, and Plenosol. All of these products are prepared from Viscum album Loranthaceae (Viscum album L. or European mistletoe) and are not available commercially in the United States.[2] Iscador is the most frequently used complementary mistletoe cancer treatment in the world, and without any promotion it has become the most widely recognized mistletoe cancer medicine in Switzerland and Germany, where 60 percent of all cancer patients are now prescribed mistletoe at some point in their treatment. It is also approved by Germany's Commission E as palliative therapy for malignant tumors (for treatment of symptoms, not as a "cure" for the disease).

Fortunately, there are very few side effects from Iscador, and it can be used in conjunction with other medications, too.[6] But proper use of Iscador requires a prescription, a doctor's supervision, and a good travel agent! For a list of Iscador treatment clinics, contact: Weleda North America by calling (800)241-1030 x5550 or visit: www.iscador.com/treatment-clinics/index.aspx

CHAPTER 9

Killing Cancer with Curcumin

After you read this chapter, you may find yourself asking for extra curry with your chicken and veggies the next time you dine out at your favorite Indian restaurant—and with very good reason. One of the main ingredients in Indian curries has had a recent boom in popularity in the West due to the ever-mounting collection of research on its health benefits—including that of a cancer blaster.

Turmeric's Healing Roots

The history of the spice turmeric, whose main active component is called curcumin, is diverse and well-documented. Curcumin is actually part of the ginger family and it is made by grinding the roots of a large-leafed Asian plant known as Curcuma Longa. The spice itself has been used by the people of India and Asia for centuries and many of its uses—from treating cuts and sores to more serious chronic diseases—are described in ancient Indian medical texts.[1]

Recently, there has been a surge in research on this spicy, golden-colored powerhouse and I've collected some especially interesting results right here for you to check out.

According to University of Chicago scientists, curcumin inhibits a cancer-provoking bacteria (H. pylori) associated with gastric and colon cancer. And biochemists in China reported in January 2007 that curcumin reduces a gene responsible for starting up prostate cancer, and could also reduce hormone receptor sensitivity to this gene.[2,3]

Curcumin also appears to be able to suppress the formation of tumors as well as protect against the DNA damage that causes cancer. One 2000 study found that the risk of tumor development in rats following exposure to X-ray dropped from 70.3 percent to 18.5 percent after receiving just 1 percent curcumin (turmeric extract) in their diet.[4]

Research done on breast cancer cells resistant to the common cancer drug Taxol showed that curcumin was also able to suppress proteins responsible for metastasis and enhance cancer cell apoptosis (pre-programmed cell death or "cell suicide")—an exciting discovery that holds great potential for cancer treatment.[5]

As a quick reminder, free radicals are byproducts of everyday

Tips for Cooking With Turmeric

- Known also as Indian saffron, turmeric is an important ingredient in curry mixes and chutneys.
- It goes well with chicken, duck, turkey, vegetables, rice, and salad dressing
- Turmeric is extremely pungent, and gets stronger when cooked
- A little goes a long way, so use it sparingly when experimenting

living and breathing, but are produced much more during exercise and exposure to smoke and chemicals. Their accumulation is largely responsible for aging and the development of health conditions such as cancer, along with other chronic diseases. Antioxidants, on the other hand, are the good guys meant to protect us from these free radicals. New research has also shown that curcumin is able to normalize antioxidant enzyme activities like superoxide dismutase (SOD) and glutathione peroxidase in the liver and blood cells of mice which means it may also hold great promise as a cancer preventative, too.[6]

A Golden Cancer Cure?

Curcumin is clearly an herbal hot topic that's already got great potential for cancer treatment, but until more human clinical trials can give us more information on its use in cancer protocols, I think curcumin is best used as part of a preventative protocol.

If you're looking to pack in a bit more curcumin than you could eat with your daily meals, you may want to consider adding it to your protocol in capsules. Here are a few companies where I found it available, but there are many out there to choose from:

Vitamin Research Products: (800)877-2447

Vitacost.com: (800)381-0759

Iherb.com: (951)616-3600

Remember to always consult with your doctor before adding anything new to your diet or supplement program.

CHAPTER 10

Ayurveda's Triumphant Cancer-Fighting Herbal Trio

"No mother?
Don't worry as long as you have Triphala"
—Indian folk saying

There's some serious wisdom in this old Indian saying about Triphala. It's been said in India that each of the three herbal fruits in the Triphala blend care for the body as a mother would care for her own child—promoting internal cleansing and removing toxins while at the same time acting as a total body tonic for improving digestion and assimilation.

Triphala is a healing powerhouse in western medical terms as well, effectively reducing cholesterol, improving circulation, reducing high blood pressure, improving liver function, and even possessing anti-inflammatory and anti-viral properties. Most recently, scientists have discovered that Triphala can slow the growth of pancreatic cancer tumors too, an amazing finding that's elevating this Ayurvedic tonic to a whole new level both in the East and the West.

Ayurveda's Golden Blend

Triphala is probably the most popular of the Ayurvedic herbal formulas, since it is not only an effective laxative with high nutritional value, but also cleanses and detoxifies without depleting the body's reserves. The blend also possesses chemical compounds called anthroquinones which help stimulate bile flow and peristalsis, the wave-like movement of the intestines. In addition, Triphala has high vitamin C content, contains linoleic oil (omega 6) as well as other important nutrients.

In 2006, scientists found that Triphala had the ability to induce cytotoxicity in tumor cells, but spares normal cells. Similarly, a December 2005 report in the *Journal of Experimental and Clinical Cancer Research* noted that Triphala was effective in reducing the incidence of tumors in and increasing the antioxidant status of animals.[1]

Another report from 2005 found that Triphala showed a significant cytotoxic (cell-killing) effect on cancer cell-lines, which may be due to the action of gallic acid, a major polyphenol in Triphala. The same authors had previously reported that Triphala "had promising antimutagenic/anticarcinogenic potential" as well, which means it could be great for blasting away cancer cells before they spread.[2]

A more recent study from the University of Pittsburgh Cancer Institute suggests that Triphala has cancer-fighting properties that prevent or slow the growth of pancreatic cancer tumors implanted in mice. This study found that Triphala caused pancreatic cancer cells to die through apoptosis, or programmed cell death (the body's normal method of disposing of damaged or unneeded cells), with no side effects. Dr. Srivastava and his colleagues found that the mice that received Triphala had increased levels of apoptosis-associated proteins and significantly smaller tumor sizes compared to the control group; Triphala-treated tumors were also half the size of tumors in untreated mice.[3]

Trying Triphala

Traditionally, Triphala is taken a tonic. You prepare it by stirring 2 or 3 grams of the powder into warm water and drinking it each evening (though you can also divide the doses and take just 1 gram two or three times a day). But be forewarned that it has a rather unique taste that not everyone loves. Luckily, it's also available in tablet or capsule form. Generally, the dose is two tablets one to three times daily or four to six tablets one time daily. You should increase or decrease the dose according to your bowel movements (meaning: cut back if you start to pass too much).

Since there are no other problems associated with using Triphala, the dose can be adjusted upwards from the suggested amount for more anti-cancer properties. Bear in mind, of course, that close monitoring by your personal health care practitioner is a must.

Triphala is available in the U.S. from a few different sources. The powder can be purchased in most Indian food import stores in larger cities and tablets are currently manufactured and distributed by Planetary Herb Formulas, Banyan Botanicals, and several other companies.[4]

With all of the amazing data emerging along with its years of use by populations in India, Triphala has definitely stood the test of time and is more than worthy of our attention as a potential addition to a cancer prevention and potential treatment protocol. Remember that even when Big Pharma tries to get its hands on herbals and boil them down to a single active compound, there are always key active components that are overlooked, which is why more often than not, herbs are best taken in their natural form. We can't put a patent on Mother Nature, and she surely knows best. I say, for now, let's sit back and enjoy Triphala as the incredible health tonic that the people of India have known and loved for centuries...

CHAPTER 11

Killing the Fungus Among Us

"The question that many people ask themselves is why, after so many years of study and research, has cancer not yet been defeated? The problem is indeed scientific, but in my opinion it is even more a problem of a cultural and social nature as it represents the very structure of knowledge at the world level—a structure that prevents that freedom of thought and creativity that is capable of finding the right solutions."

—Dr. Tullio Simoncini[1]

Could you imagine a cure for cancer sitting right in your own kitchen cupboard? If you ask oncologist Dr. Tullio Simoncini from Rome, Italy, he'll tell you exactly that—that tumors can be completely dissolved with the power of a compound that's a fixture in almost every pantry: plain old sodium bicarbonate, also known as baking soda.

We've known for years that sodium bicarbonate can kill all sorts of fungi and microorganisms, and in the early 1990s Dr. Simoncini discovered that it can neutralize tumor masses, too. In fact, for the last 15 years, sodium bicarbonate treatment has helped hundreds of patients overcome various forms of cancer. Even better, the treatment is incredibly inexpensive and has no side effects. So why haven't we heard more about this remarkable breakthrough?

Well, based on what you've read so far, you've probably guessed that where there are no big bucks to be earned, Big Pharma's back is sharply turned. But lucky for us, word is spreading about sodium bicarbonate treatment, and it's already available in some clinics in the USA, offering a ray of light in the cancer fight.

Candida Acts as Cancer Glue

In his scientific research, Dr. Simoncini found that all solid cancers are bound together by a fungus, which produces an acid-based glue that holds cancer cells together. The name of that fungus? None other than Candida albicans, the common cause of many yeast infections.

Specifically, Dr. Simoncini found out that Candida plays a vital role in cancer's ability to survive, by making toxins that impair a cell's ability to self-destruct while allowing mutated cells to replicate into full-blown cancer. When Candida becomes intertwined with tumors, it stays alive along with the cancer. So, according to Dr. Simoncini, the trick to destroying cancer is to blast away the fungus that supports it.

Now, you would think that if it's as simple as a yeast infection, then doctors should be able to knock it out with an anti-fungal drug, right? Unfortunately, according to Dr. Simoncini, it's not quite that simple.

Since the era of antibiotics began, fungi have literally been forgotten to the point where not only is our technology lacking accurate testing for fungal infections, but Candida is also resistant to our anti-fungal drugs.[2]

The Cancer-Fungus Connection

There's some interesting research out there to support Dr. Simoncini's Candida-cancer theory, too. For example, the late Milton White, M.D., who believed that cancer is a "chronic, intracellular, infectious, biologically induced spore (fungus) transformation disease," found fungus in *every sample of cancer tissue that he studied.* In addition, just a few years back, in 1999, Meinolf Karthaus, M.D., saw three different children with leukemia suddenly go into remission after getting a megadose of a triple antifungal drug cocktail.[3,4]

You're probably wondering where all of this fungus comes from. Well, to figure out what's going on inside our bodies, I believe it's always smartest to first take a look at what we're putting in them. And surely the typical American diet is far from ideal. In fact, most American diets are based on foods that Candida just love to feast on. In addition, certain refined grains are commonly contaminated with cancer-causing fungal poisons which can make the problem

Top 10 Ways to Kick Candida: Foods to Avoid

- refined sugar
- white bread and pastries
- mushrooms and yeast
- aged cheeses
- cold cuts and preserved meats
- peanuts and roasted nuts
- condiments like ketchup and mustard
- alcoholic beverages
- melons or excessive amounts of any fruit
- all leftovers

worse.[5] Of course, antibiotics also play a big role in welcoming Candida, since they destroy the normal, protective bacteria that live in the gut, allowing intestinal yeast and fungi to grow unchecked. All of this can lead to immune suppression, symptoms of any autoimmune disease, or even cancer.

The $3 Cancer Cure

So what, you ask, does the baking soda in my kitchen cabinet have to do with Candida? Well, according to Dr. Simoncini, all cancerous tumors are highly acidic and lack oxygen, mainly a result of fungus activity in the body that has gotten out of control. Baking soda is what chemists call a base, and it has the powerful ability to neutralize a highly acidic tumor mass, and stop tumor growth. Sodium bicarbonate administered directly to a neoplastic mass by injection into selected arteries leading to the site of the tumor destroys the fungal colonies living in it, stopping tumor growth without negatively affecting the rest of you.[6]

According to Dr. Simoncini, an at-home, ingestible version of baking soda treatment can be used (with the supervision of your doctor, of course) in certain types of cancer limited to a particular organ (i.e., it should not be affecting the surrounding tissue), such as the mouth, esophagus, stomach, intestine, and rectum. If you want to try it, be sure to use only an aluminum-free baking soda like Bob's Red Mill or a pharmaceutical grade. Take 1 teaspoon of baking soda with a glass of water in the morning and 1 in the evening every day for one month.[7]

In all other cases, though, you should opt for the infusions mentioned above—and the assistance of a doctor is *mandatory* for these. But while it's a bit more involved than the at-home version of baking soda therapy, Dr. Simoncini has reported that many cases of brain, bladder, breast, spleen, liver, lung, prostate, stomach, pancreatic, and other cancers have resolved with the IV treatment. In general, he has found that if the fungi are sensitive to the sodium bicarbonate and the tumor size is below 3 cm, the response will be around 90 percent. In terminal cases, the response is around 50 percent when the patient is in reasonable condition (for more advanced terminal patients it is of course a smaller percentage).[8]

The Simoncini treatment protocol involves 500 cc of a 5 percent bicarbonate solution given intravenously over one hour, six days a week, or in the case of localized, accessible tumors (like those found in breast cancer), the solution can be injected directly at the site. Many of Dr. Simoncini's colleagues have modified his protocol to include alternating weeks of bicarbonate with infusions of high-dose intravenous vitamin C six days a week. Amazingly, many have found that this approach only takes six weeks to get rid of many cancers.[7]

I believe there's some good science behind Dr. Simoncini's treatment and don't see any harm in alkalinizing the body a bit with some sodium bicarbonate. There are several clinics out there which offer this treatment. To learn more about one of these clinics, visit www.camelotcancercare.com.

Of course, as with every treatment in this book, do consult with your doctor before implementing any new treatment.

CHAPTER 12

The "Long Life" Diet for Beating Cancer

Macrobiotic literally means "long life" in Ancient Greek. Since the time of Hippocrates, philosophers and physicians from many parts of the world have used the term to signify living in harmony with nature. The philosophy of macrobiotics is based on the idea of achieving balance. Years later, in the 1930s, a Japanese philosopher named George Ohsawa developed a diet protocol based on these principles.

Ohsawa believed that macrobiotic diets could cure cancer and other serious illnesses by attempting to balance the excess Yin and Yang energies in a person's life, which he asserted are at the foundation of many different types of cancer. Although the macrobiotic dietary guidelines are only one aspect of a larger philosophical and spiritual system, it's the diet part that's drawn the most attention in the West.(1)

Its popularity in the U.S. began in the 1960s but the diet really came to center stage in the 1980s, when a physician and president of Philadelphia Hospital, Anthony Sattilaro, published a book about how following a macrobiotic diet helped him beat prostate cancer. Since then, macrobiotic diets have been used by hundreds of people to treat cancer.

Back to Basics

Like other anti-cancer diets, the macrobiotic diet is based on dietary principles of simplicity and avoidance of "toxins" that come from eating dairy products, meats, and oily foods.

The standard macrobiotic diet today consists of:

- 50 to 60 percent organically grown whole grains
- 20 to 25 percent locally and organically grown fruits and vegetables
- 5 to 10 percent soups made with vegetables, seaweed, grains, beans, and miso (a fermented soy product)

Other elements of the diet include occasional helpings of fresh, white-meat fish, nuts, seeds, pickles, Asian condiments, and non-stimulating and non-aromatic teas.

The diet excludes vegetables such as potatoes, tomatoes, eggplant, peppers, asparagus, spinach, beets, zucchini, and avocados and advises against eating fruits that do not grow locally, such as bananas, pineapples, and other tropical fruits. The use of dairy products, eggs, coffee, sugar, stimulant and aromatic herbs, red meat, poultry, and processed foods is also discouraged.

The macrobiotic philosophy also says that fluid intake should be governed by thirst and then only teas made from roasted grains, dandelion greens, or the cooking water of soba noodles are generally considered acceptable. Drinking and cooking water must be purified and there are specific guidelines for cooking food, along with rules

Some Macro Extras

- Macrobiotic dieters do not cook with microwaves or electricity, nor do they consume vitamin or mineral supplements, or heavily processed foods.
- Macrobiotic food is always chewed until it is fluid in order to help with digestion and since food is thought to be sacred, it is always prepared in a peaceful setting.
- To maintain proper yin/yang balance, all extremely "yang" foods and all extremely "yin" foods should be avoided. All animal foods, including eggs and dairy products, are believed to have a strong yang quality. Extremely yin foods and beverages include refined sugars, chocolate, tropical fruits, soda, fruit juice, coffee, and hot spices.
- In addition, all foods processed with artificial colors, flavors, or preservatives must be avoided.
- According to macrobiotic proponents, living within the natural order means eating only what is necessary for one's condition and desires, and learning to adjust in a peaceful way to life's changes.[3]

about what types of pots, pans, and utensils should be used.[2]

We already know, based on a number of population-based studies, that a low-fat, plant-based diet using whole grains, legumes, vegetables, and fruit is the healthiest for cancer prevention and preventing cancer recurrence. Though the therapeutic benefits of macrobiotic diets haven't been studied extensively, they do encompasses many of these elements. And proponents of the diet often point to the results of a 1993 study involving patients with pancreatic cancer where 52 percent of those who followed a macrobiotic diet were still alive after one year, compared to only 10 percent of those who made no dietary changes.[4]

Another piece of interesting evidence in favor of macrobiotics is the population-based study which reported that cancer of the lung, breast, and colon increased two to three times among Japanese women between 1950 and 1975. During that period, milk consumption increased 15-fold, meat, eggs, and poultry consumption rose seven and a half times and rice consumption dropped by 70 percent.[5]

Here's a quick outline of some of the foods you would include in a macrobiotic diet:

- Whole grains: brown rice, barley, millet, oats, corn, rye, whole wheat, and buckwheat. These are believed to be the most balanced foods on the yin/yang continuum. Only small portions of pasta and bread from refined flour may be eaten.
- Fresh vegetables: cabbage, broccoli, cauliflower, kale, bok choy, collards, mustard greens, turnips, turnip greens, onion, daikon radish, acorn squash, butternut squash, and pumpkin. Vegetables to be eaten occasionally (two to three times per week) include celery, iceberg lettuce, mushrooms, snow peas, and string beans. Up to 1/3 of the total vegetable intake can be raw. Otherwise, vegetables should be lightly steamed, boiled, baked, or sautéed with a small amount of unrefined cooking oil (preferably corn or sesame).
- Beans and sea vegetables: adzuki beans, chickpeas (garbanzo beans), lentils, and tofu. Sea vegetables, including wakame, hijiki, kombu, and nori, are rich in many vitamins and minerals, and are typi-

cally a part of each meal.

- Soups and broths: soups containing miso (soy bean paste), vegetables, and beans are acceptable.
- Nuts and seeds: include a few servings each week in moderation. Seeds and nuts can be lightly roasted and salted with sea salt or shoyu.
- Fresh fish: halibut, flounder, cod, or sole are permissible. Fish or seafood are eaten with horseradish, wasabi, ginger, mustard, or grated daikon to help the body detoxify the chemicals in them (see the sidebar on page 76).
- Fruit: local fruit can be consumed several times a week, including apples, pears, peaches, apricots, grapes, berries, melons, and other fruit. Tropical fruit such as mango, pineapple, and papaya is usually avoided.
- Desserts: naturally sweet foods such as apples, squash, adzuki beans, and dried fruit. Natural sweeteners such as rice syrup, barley malt, and amazake can be used in moderation, approximately two to three times per week. Sugar, honey, molasses, chocolate, carob, and other sweeteners are avoided.
- Oils: one of the most common oils used is dark sesame oil. Other oils that are recommended are light sesame oil, corn oil, and mustard seed oil.
- Soy: tofu and other soy based products. Proponents of the diet say that the high phytoes-

trogens in the foods may help to balance female hormones and prevent breast cancer but the jury is still out on how much soy we should be eating these days, so don't overdo it.

- Condiments and seasonings: natural sea salt, shoyu, brown rice vinegar, umeboshi vinegar, umeboshi plums, grated ginger root, fermented pickles, gomashio (roasted sesame seeds), roasted seaweed, and sliced scallions.[6]

Eating Your Way to a Long, Cancer-free Life

Although the studies are few and far between, we can be pretty sure that a plant-based macrobiotic diet is preferable to the high-saturated-fat, refined-sugar-filled, processed-meat-laden standard

Go Fish

Some people following macrobiotic diets consume fish on occasion, but due to the toxic chemicals in fish and shellfish (found at concentrations as high as 9 million times the levels in the polluted water in which they swim), it's probably best for cancer patients to avoid fish altogether.

Mercury (which occurs in especially high levels in tuna and swordfish) and pesticides, such as DDT, PCBs, and dioxin, have been linked to cancers and many other health problems. Avoiding fish eliminates half of all mercury exposure and reduces intake of other toxins as well. I'd suggest that if you choose to follow a macrobiotic diet, stick with a plant-based diet along with the other lifestyle guidelines.[8]

American fare. Macrobiotic diets emphasize foods that tend to be lacking in the North American diet such as fiber-rich whole grains, vegetables, and beans.

It's important to mention, though, that the diet is restrictive and may be lacking in certain nutrients, such as protein, vitamin B12, iron, magnesium, and calcium, so if you decide to try this diet, keep an eye on your energy levels and if they dip to low, consult with your doctor or nutritionist.

As those of you who know my philosophy are aware, I'm very much an advocate of nutrient supplementation. However, much of that stance is based on the fact that our Standard American Diet (SAD) is so woefully deficient (and chemical-packed), that supplements are far more necessary than in a diet built on the premise that everything must be natural, close-to-home, not microwaved, etc. Though I'm still a dyed-in-the-wool "vitamin nut," for those who are not, it's worth being aware of the macrobiotic approach.

CHAPTER 13

Nature's Secret Cancer-Fighting Vitamin

Over 150 years ago, two French chemists discovered a natural compound in bitter almonds and certain fruit pits which would become the source of one of the most controversial alternative cancer treatments to date.

Laetrile, also known as amygdalin, originates from the seeds of plants in the Prunus rosacea family and has been used to cure cancer for centuries. In fact, it dates way back to the Ancient Chinese who used it in its natural form by consuming bitter almonds to cure tumors.

Scientific studies have since revealed that this incredible compound is actually able to kill cancer cells while keeping healthy cells unharmed, using selective toxicity—something chemo and radiation cannot do. Even more incredible is that doctors who treat their patients with Laetrile boast a near 100 percent recovery rate.

Although Laetrile has been the subject of numerous studies which have proven its great efficacy in fighting cancer, in the early 1980s, the NCI launched a vicious attack of propaganda against it. As a result, it was never submitted for FDA approval, nor is it available anymore in the United States. But it is still available in Mexico and thousands with cancer who have been told they have only months to live flock there each year to receive their Laetrile therapy. And, believe it or not, *many have recovered and are now living normal lives.*

Much to the dismay of the American Medical Association (AMA) and the other cancer organizations who tried to pull the rug from underneath Laetrile and dub it a fraud, this amazing treatment continues to be a blessing for the many who have made Laetrile their weapon of choice against cancer—and won.

Seeds of History

Amygdalin was first used as an anticancer treatment in Russia back in 1845, but its first recorded use for treating cancer in the United States was in the early 1920s. Shortly afterwards, the formula was deemed "too toxic" by the medical establishment, and amygdalin was abandoned. Luckily, years later—in the 1950s—the compound resurfaced and was dubbed "Laetrile" by the father-son team of Ernest T. Krebs Sr., M.D., and E.T. Krebs Jr. (Laetrile is actually a contraction of the more formal name of purified Amygdalin: laevo-mandelonitrile-glucoside.)

The Krebses found Laetrile to be a member of a group of chemicals called nitrilosides, also sometimes called vitamin B17. These compounds are essentially non-toxic and are found in many edible plants.[1]

The Krebs team theorized that vitamin B17 plays a critical role in keeping the human body free from cancer. In other words, they believed that B17 deficiency is the root cause of cancer, similar to how vitamin C deficiency causes the disease scurvy. But just as someone with scurvy requires higher amounts of vitamin C even after the disease has gone away, so the Krebses also asserted that Laetrile was not a cure for cancer, but rather a form of *cancer control* which would need to be taken indefinitely, even after the original cancer went away.[1]

The Truth Behind the Controversy

The way Laetrile works in the body is actually a big part of the controversy that surrounds it. You see, Laetrile molecules actually contain cyanide. In fact, that's what kills the cancer. When Laetrile meets up with a cancer cell, the cancer cell's major enzyme combines with it and causes a chemical reaction that releases the cyanide and kills the cancer cell. Many opponents of Laetrile will tell you that the cyanide it contains can be very dangerous—even deadly. But the truth is, the cyanide is only deadly to cancerous cells.

In fact, when Laetrile comes into contact with normal, healthy cells they release an enzyme that breaks it down into two byproducts which are actually beneficial and even help your body produce vitamin B12. And any excess of these byproducts is expelled from the body via the kidneys.

This process is known as selective toxicity, which means that Laetrile can select which cells it wants to kill.[2]

It *is* important, however to avoid taking probiotics when taking Laetrile orally, since these good bacteria can sometimes make this conversion to cyanide if taken in excess.[3]

B17 Backed by Research

The evidence in favor of Laetrile as an effective cancer treatment comes from three different sets of research data: epidemiological, animal tests, and human clinical use by experienced doctors.

The epidemiological, or population-based, evidence for Laetrile comes from tribes such as those in West Pakistan, the aboriginal Eskimaux, and the tribes of South Africa and South America, where cancer tends to be rare compared to the high rates present in America and Europe. These indigenous populations live on a native diet based on fruits and vegetables which contains as much as 250 to 3,000 mg of nitrilosides (the same family of chemical compounds that Laetrile is a member of) in a daily ration. To put that into perspective, the diets you and I are used to in the West provide more like an average of 2 mg of nitrilosides a day. While we don't know for sure whether the Laetrile can be credited with the vibrant health of the indigenous people in the areas listed above, there's definitely much more nitriloside consumption going on with these folks, and there's no question anyway that a diet rich in fruits and vegetables, including those rich in Laetrile, and the nutrients they pack, are an essential part of beating any cancer.(4)

The animal studies on Laetrile have some clearer evidence on its anti-cancer effect. In 1977, Dr. Vern L. van Breeman at Salisbury State College, Maryland, added apricot kernels (which are naturally rich in Laetrile) to the standard food of mice bred to develop breast cancer and leukemia. They found that these mice had increased survival times as opposed to those that did not get the Laetrile in their diets. When Dr. van Breeman reported his early findings, seven of the animals in the leukemia control group and five in the breast cancer control group had died, while none of the mice eating the apricot kernels had. In fact, the leukemia-prone mice that ate apricot kernels lived up to 50 percent longer than would normally be expected.(5)

Yet another study found that Laetrile more than doubled the survival time for patients with inoperable lung cancer. And, in a third study, Laetrile injected into lab animals in dosages of 500 mg/kg resulted in a 70 percent increase in survival time compared to the controls.(6)

Foods that Naturally Contain Laetrile

The Mexican doctors using Laetrile in their practices say that eating a diet high in B17 will help keep cancer at bay. Here's a list of the top Laetrile foods:

- Fruit Seeds: apple seeds, millet seeds, plum kernels, apricot kernels, cherry kernels, peach kernels
- Berries: blackberries, boysenberries cranberries, currants, gooseberries, huckleberries, raspberries, strawberries
- Grains: brown rice, buckwheat, millet, barley
- Nuts and Seeds: cashews, flax seeds, macadamia nuts, pecans, walnuts, bitter almond
- Beans: fava beans, garbanzo beans, lentils, lima beans, mung beans
- Vegetables: spinach, alfalfa, watercress, yams, beet tops, bamboo shoots
- Other: sorghum cane syrup, brewer's yeast[7]

The Big B17 Cover-Up

Perhaps the most important studies on Laetrile come from veteran cancer researcher, Kanematsu Sugiura of the Sloan Kettering Institute, who performed three sets of experiments on Laetrile between September 1972 and June 1973 on mice with mammary tumors. Ralph Moss, who was the assistant director of public affairs at Sloan Kettering at the time, recalled that

> *"Kanematsu Sugiura...astonished me when he told me he was working on Laetrile (B17), at the time it was the most controversial thing in cancer.... We in public affairs were giving out statements that*

> *Laetrile was worthless, it was quackery, and people should not abandon proven therapies....He took down lab books and showed me that in fact, Laetrile is dramatically effective in stopping the spread of cancer. The animals were genetically programmed to get breast cancer and about 80-90% of them normally get spread of the cancer from the breast to the lungs which is a common route in humans also, for how people die of breast cancer, and instead when they gave the animals Laetrile by injection only 10-20% of them got lung metastases. And these facts were verified by many people, including the pathology department."*

When he concluded his studies, Suguira released an internal report to his colleagues at Sloan-Kettering that said *"the results clearly show that Amygdalin significantly inhibits the appearance of lung metastases in mice bearing spontaneous mammary tumors and increases significantly the inhibition of the growth of the primary tumor over the appearance of inhibition in the untreated animals."*

But not surprisingly, these results weren't to the liking of the big dogs at Sloan-Kettering, who suppressed the true results. In 1982 the results of Phase I and II trials on Laetrile involving 178 patients with advanced cancers were published in the New England Journal of Medicine and Laetrile was officially labeled there as "ineffective" as a treatment for cancer.

And when Ralph Moss held a press conference to publicize the suppressed results of the Laetrile studies, he was fired the next day for "failing to carry out his most basic job responsibility."[2,8,9]

With Moss gone, the "ineffective" label stuck. And in 1974, the American Cancer Society officially labeled Laetrile as "quackery." But advocates for Laetrile still dispute this label and claim that financial motivations tainted the research—something we've unfortunately come across time and time again in the world of cancer treatments.

Laetrile advocates pointed out that 66 percent of the patients selected for the trial had already been subjected to toxic chemotherapy, which can negate the effects of Laetrile. Critics of the NEJM study also questioned the quality of the Laetrile used in the trial. Some reports even claim that the substance used in the study didn't contain any Amygdalin at all! In an effort to ensure a proper trial, one of the clinics using Laetrile had even offered to provide free treatments for the study. But the offer was refused.

So while Laetrile is currently used as an anticancer treatment all over the world, it is not approved in the United States as a treatment for cancer. In fact, the FDA actually seeks jail sentences for vendors selling Laetrile as a cancer treatment, calling it a "highly toxic product that has not shown any effect on treating cancer."

However, in certain U.S. states the use of Laetrile is authorized for purposes other than treating cancer. In Montana, a doctor may actually prescribe it as a dietary supplement to a patient not suffering from a known disease or illness, while in Indiana a physician who has signed a written informed request can prescribe or administer Amygdalin in place of, or as an adjunct to, accepted therapies for the treatment of a malignancy, a disease, an illness, or a physical condition of a patient. But for outright Laetrile cancer treatment, your best bet is to travel to one of the hospitals in Mexico where it's given regularly, such as the Oasis of Hope Hospital (888-500-HOPE; www.oasisofhope.com).

If you're interested in learning more about Laetrile therapy, I suggest reading *The Ultimate Guide to B17 Metabolic Therapy.*[10]

More Secrets to Laetrile's Success

Many practitioners who treat with Laetrile recommend the use of certain nutrients that are necessary for Laetrile to work properly. These include zinc, vitamin C, manganese, magnesium, selenium, vitamin A, vitamin E, vitamin B6, vitamin B12, and folic acid. Pancreatic or proteolytic enzymes are also a typical addition to the Laetrile protocol, but it's essential that you seek guidance from a practitioner who is a Laetrile expert before beginning the treatment and supplements for specific dosages.

CHAPTER 14 An Endangered Medicine from the Taiwanese Mountains

Unless you live in Taiwan, you've probably never even heard of Antrodia camphorata. I certainly hadn't—which took me by surprise, considering the fact that cancer-fighting mushrooms like this one are such a hot topic in natural medicine these days. But in the course of my research, the reasons for its obscurity became clear as day. Like a lot of the cures I've shared with you, there's a big catch.

You see, this particular mushroom is practically extinct. So why am I telling you about a cure that you may never get your hands on? Well, with the sweeping advances in cultivating technologies over the past decade, scientists at Taipei's Well Shine Biotechnology Development have discovered a way to grow this mushroom in mass and unlike those who have tried before them, they've produced a product that is nearly a perfect genetic match (99.97 percent, to be exact) to wild Antrodia camphorata.

The Price of Protecting this Miracle Healer

Antrodia camphorata grows in the remote Taiwanese mountainside, as high as 1,500 meters above sea level, where the upper branches of the slow-growing Cinnamomum kanehirai Hay tree are its sole hosts. But this fungi's towering natural habitat isn't the only thing that makes it nearly impossible to find—the Hay tree also happens to yield the best-quality lumber in the country. So much so, in fact, that the fragile species is now teetering toward extinction—a trend that led to its current protected status, which the Taiwanese government put into place 25 years ago. Today, in Taiwan, harvesting this wild cancer miracle at the expense of its endangered host is criminal and it therefore comes as no surprise that specimens of the mushroom are so rare that they sell for the equivalent of $600 an ounce.

But it hasn't always been so rare.

It was 1773 when the famous Chinese doctor Wu-Sha arrived at Formosa, the main island of Taiwan. At the time, many local inhabitants were plagued by alcoholism, and Dr. Wu immediately observed unusually high incidence of headaches, hepatitis, cirrhosis, and other complications of the disease. But more perplexing was the swiftness with which the Formosans recovered—an anomaly that, he would later discover, was directly linked to the peoples' reliance on Antrodia camphorata.

Dr. Wu's future studies revealed that Antrodia camphorata was far more effective than any of the other herbs typically used in Traditional Chinese Medicine—especially against pain, bacterial infections, poisons, liver failure, and cancer.

With this lengthy folk history, it's a wonder that the mushroom's scientific name wasn't even confirmed until 1997—and that the majority of formal studies on this mushroom have only been performed in the last 10 years. But despite its slow start, research on Antrodia camphorata continues to pick up steam. In fact, I dug up lots of studies documenting its powerful effects against conditions like inflammation and toxicity—and most notably, its ability to target, revert, and even destroy cancer cells.

A Taiwanese Cancer Wipeout

The first published studies on Antrodia camphorata came in the early 2000s, and most primarily demonstrated the extract's anti-oxidant and liver-protecting qualities. In one study, researchers from Taipei Medical University compared preparations of Antrodia camphorata to an isolated flavonoid found in milk thistle called silymarin, a popular treatment for liver toxicity and cirrhosis. Results showed that the mushroom stood up to the powerful flavonoid and offered significant liver protection to mice that were treated with it—most likely, the scientists theorized, due to its strong free radical scavenging abilities.[1]

Later research served as further confirmation for these early findings—only in these instances, studies revealed that the extract wasn't just preventing liver damage, but was actually inducing apoptosis in several human liver cancer lines and inhibiting cancer cell growth.[2,3] But liver cancer cells weren't the only ones that extracts of Antrodia camphorata stood up to in the laboratory.

Research conducted as recently as 2008 has shown that this fungus can not only prevent metastasis in bladder cancer cell lines[4], breast cancer cell lines[5], leukemia cell lines[6], and lung cancer cell lines[7]—it can even reverse and obliterate them.

The mechanism for Antrodia's unparalleled healing powers, scientists propose, is its remarkably high composition of naturally occurring polysaccharides, adenosine, chitin, superoxide dismutase, vitamins—and an especially huge quantity of cancer-fighting plant compounds called triterpenoids. The popular medicinal mushroom Ganoderma lucidum, for example, boasts about 20 to 50 different forms of this particular compound (at a total content of about 1 to 3 percent). But chemical analysis shows that Antrodia camphorata contains over 200 different kinds of triterpenoids, resulting in a total content of about 20 to 45 percent—that's nearly 50 times greater.

A Miracle Mushroom With Only One Source

This research is just a small sampling of what's out there—so it's easy to see why Antrodia camphorata's widening availability, both in the U.S. and abroad, is such a huge breakthrough. And with all of this hard science, it's only a matter of time before the market is flooded with versions of the mushroom, right? Well, not exactly.

According to Roland Li, from the Khong Guan Corporation—also the man who spearheaded this product's U.S. launch, there are two ways to produce fungus in a laboratory. Using a liquid medium (aqua-culture), you can replicate the mushroom's mycelium (a web-like structure on which the actual fruit grows) but not the fruit itself. Earlier attempts at reproducing the elusive mushroom usually took this form. With this method, however, it's far too difficult to yield an amount suitable for mass production and sale—much less a product with the amount of triterpenoids necessary to make for a bonafide natural cancer killer.

But this problem has been solved with the innovation of "solid-culturing"—a process that Well Shine Development has perfected. In this case, scientists grow the actual fruiting body of the mushroom. And when matched with a pristinely controlled environment, the result is a product that is the closest thing available to wild Antrodia camphorata —in triterpenoid content, and consequently, disease-fighting capacity too.

Well Shine is the only company in the world to have mastered the patented culturing technique and after extensive toxicity and safety testing, we now have access to the same supplement successfully used as a complementary cancer therapy in Taiwan for almost a decade now. Their product, called Vitalsil, is 100 percent solid-cultured Antrodia camphorata, and it's now being imported exclusively by Khong Guan Corporation.

I'll end with one word of caution—and it's one that you might have already guessed by now: Vitalsil's price is on the steep side. The recommended dosage is two to three capsules one to four times a day—and at $138 per 60-capsule bottle, you could be shelling out quite a bit to include this mushroom in your daily supplement regimen. But the effects may be well worth the cost.

CHAPTER 15

The Poisonous Plant Killing Cancer

Despite being known to many as one of the most poisonous plants around, oleander has actually been used for centuries as a potent herbal medicine to heal a variety of health conditions. And in the 1970s, the famous plant took on a new role in Turkey, when Dr. Huseyin Ozel discovered he could treat advanced and inoperable cancer with it. Again and again, Dr. Ozel treated cancer cases that were pronounced terminal and with no hope for recovery, and gave people a new chance at life with the help of oleander extract.

After further research and scientific presentations to the medical community, Dr. Ozel even took out a patent on the plant, and called it Anvirzel with the hopes of making it available to the world. Ironically, though, it was Dr. Ozel's great success that led to long periods of controversy from the Turkish medical establishment, and many even tagged him a charlatan.

But when scores of patients rose up to testify about how they had been cured with oleander extract when all other treatment options had failed, the truth of Dr. Ozel's successes prevailed. Of course, the FDA feels very differently about Oleander—but today, this remedy is available and thriving outside the U.S. as a viable treatment for cancer, vouching again for wonders and incredible staying power of Mother Nature.

Ancient Folk Remedy

The name "oleander" refers to two plant species, Nerium oleander (common oleander) and Thevetia peruviana (yellow oleander), which both grow in temperate climates throughout the world. The plant has a long history. In the 15th century BC, the Mesopotamians knew of the healing properties of oleander and the Babylonians used a mixture of oleander and licorice to treat hangovers. Pliny the Elder of ancient Greece wrote about the appearance and properties of oleander, and Arab physicians were the first to use oleander as a cancer treatment in the 8th century AD.

Dr. Huseyin Ozel first discovered the plant's use when he observed local villagers in Turkey who lived in high altitudes, drinking an oleander folk remedy against leukemia. Feeling he had determined the cause of the villager's good health, Dr. Ozel became intrigued with the plant and began to prepare and work with various extracts of oleander himself in 1966 while he was the head of the surgical department at Mugla State Hospital of Turkey.[1]

Dr. O's Oleander Studies

Once he'd conducted animal sturies that determined the toxicology and effects of Nerium oleander extract (or NOE), Dr. Ozel conducted further experiments and developed his treatment until he eventually began tests on terminal human cases (by law, he could not treat patients with an experimental drug, such as NOE, unless they had exhausted all other conventional treatment methods with no response or were diagnosed as advanced stage, terminal cases).

After initial success in treating human cancer patients with NOE, Dr. Ozel began to discuss his findings with other professionals in his field, and sought analysis of the extract from Turkish laboratories to understand the empirical results, but they were unable to characterize the extracted compounds.

At a medical conference where he presented his findings, the response from the scientific community was weak, to say the least. Their skepticism was mainly due to the fact that Dr. Ozel's presentation contradicted what little literature there was on the oleander species. However, Dr. Ozel was undaunted by the lack of support for the ideas presented and continued his research as patients continued to seek treatment.

Tests performed in Europe in 1986 and 1987 proved the effect of NOE on the immune system as well as cancer. In fact, these studies showed that it was at least six times as potent as the most active commercially available immune-stimulants. In 1988, a research team was formed at Munich University Pharmacology Institute to isolate the active components contained in NOE, and several compounds were identified that might be responsible for some part of the immune activity.

In July 1990, the initial results were presented at the symposium of Biology and Chemistry of Active Natural Substances (BACANS) which was held in Bonn, Germany. Interestingly, no single component of the extract was found to be the sole source of oleander's benefits. Instead, its benefits are induced by a complex mixture of components in the extract, acting together or synergistically, to balance the immune system.[1]

The Long Journey Toward Approval

Dr. Ozel soon took out a patent on NOE, calling it Anvirzel. Unfortunately, since Ozel had claimed that oleander was a cure for cancer, and since his extract was patented and given a trademark, the FDA considers oleander an "unproven medicine." And because of the toxicity of the raw oleander plant, NOE must have it's safety and effectiveness proven before the FDA will allow it's use even as an herbal supplement.

Today, the lengthy and costly three-phase FDA trial process for approval of Anvirzel or any other oleander extract has a long way to go, although millions of investor dollars are counting on it ultimately being approved. In 2000, Ozelle Pharmaceuticals had successful phase I FDA trials conducted on Anvirzel, but ran into financial problems and had to reorganize.

The bottom line is that it could be years, if ever, before an oleander-based medicine gets FDA approval due to the fact is that it takes hundreds of millions of dollars to get a new drug successfully through all the FDA trials.[1]

But another company, Phoenix Biotech, has obtained a patent for Anvirzel in Honduras and for the past eight years, the Salud Integral clinic in that country has successfully treated numerous patients (many of whom travel from the U.S.) with it.

Studies are Still Going Strong

I recently found some newer research on oleander, which only strengthens the case for its growing anti-cancer reputation. In a 2000 study, it was found that the NOE Anvirzel induces cell death in human cancer cells.[2] Another study published recently in peer-reviewed journals showed that an aqueous extract of the oleander plant induced and increased autophagy in pancreatic cancer cells. Autophagy is a process in which a cell destroys proteins and other substances in its cytoplasm (the fluid inside the cell membrane but outside the nucleus), which may lead to cell death, as in the study with pancreatic cancer cells.[3]

So, we basically can say that oleander helps to treat cancer by:

- Boosting the immune system
- Causing apoptosis, or normal cell death, in cancer cells
- Enhancing autophagic cancer cell death (as tested on pancreatic cancer cells)

Oleander also enhances chemo and radiation and when used along with either one, and it either eliminates or greatly lessens all known side effects of chemo and those of radiation (with the exception being hair loss when the chemo drug of choice is Cisplatin).

Two Ways to Take Oleander

There are two ways to take oleander as a treatment for cancer. Let me stress, though, that the preferred way is to take it as a capsule or extract. These versions have already been formulated to be at a safe level for humans, but are toxic to cancer cells.[4] But, if you like, you can make your own oleander remedy, known as "oleander soup" at home (see page 99 for recipe). Either way, before you decide, it is imperative that you consult with your doctor first before beginning to take oleander.

If you do decide to take Oleander soup, begin with ¼ to ½ of a teaspoon two or three times a day after meals. Work your dose up slowly, a week at a time, until you reach 1 tablespoon three times a day after meals.

Side effects are normally fairly mild, especially when compared to standard chemo or radiation therapy side effects, and vary from one individual to another. In fact, some people don't experience side effects at all. But when they do occur, they typically include mild fever, headache, diarrhea, nausea, and sometimes vomiting. Usually these effects go away in a couple of weeks, as the body adjusts to the oleander soup. After a month or so, perhaps less, you should be up to tolerating the full dose (1 tablespoon, three times per day) with minimum reaction. But remember, once a disease like cancer is stopped, it can return so you might want to think about continuing smaller maintenance dosages.(1)

A Few More Words of Caution on Oleander

Raw oleander plant is extremely toxic. But there have been no verified reports of serious adverse reactions or side-effects due to properly prepared oleander extract taken according to directions. Still, oleander soup should only be used under medical supervision, preferably that of someone well-versed in herbal and integrative medicine.(1)

Most herbs can be taken with oleander, however, because oleander makes your heart work harder, you should avoid herbs that contain cardiac glycosides or that have blood thinning properties. Likewise, oleander is compatible with virtually all medicines and chemo, the only exceptions being digitalis and blood thinning agents such as Warfarin and Coumadin.

It is important to stress that anyone who makes the home version should make absolutely certain that the plant(s) they use have not been contaminated with pesticides or other chemicals. If you feel a tingling or numbing sensation when the extract is touched to your lips, it is a sign of contamination (most likely by the pesticide Malathion).

Soup's On!

Making oleander soup is a delicate process, and to ensure your safety, it's absolutely critical that you follow the steps outlined below EXACTLY.

1. Wear rubber gloves. Any part of the plant can be used, but trimming the new growth 6 to 8 inches from the tips will ensure that the plant lives. Avoid touching the cut ends of the plant and be sure to wear thick rubber gloves (without them, the sap will penetrate skin and is toxic).
2. Place the plant trimmings into a large stainless steel pot.
3. Fill the pot with water, completely covering trimmings. Pack the oleander down into the water, making sure the water level is at least two inches from the top, so it won't boil over.
4. Place the lid on the pot and cook the oleander at a slow, rolling boil with the lid on for 3.5 to 4 hours.
5. Remove plant material with tongs and discard carefully.
6. Boil the remaining liquid again for another 2 to 3 hours, reducing the liquid to about 30 percent of what was originally in the pot. (It should be about the same consistency as chicken soup broth.)
7. Keeping the pot covered, let the remaining liquid cool for about 2 hours until it reaches room temperature.
8. Line four plastic colanders with a layer of paper towels, then stack each of the colanders on top of one another and place a 2-quart pan or bowl underneath.
9. Once the broth is cool, use a soup ladle to slowly pour the it into the stacked, lined colanders.
10. Change the paper towel filters in each of the colanders and then repeat the filtering process one more time.
11. To preserve the end product, mix it with 80 proof vodka or apple cider vinegar (organic non-distilled is by far the best) in a 50/50 ratio. This will extend its shelf life by at least six months.
12. Using a funnel, pour the mixture into 20-oz. bottles (you can use empty plastic water bottles, though brown glass bottles are a bit better). Screw the caps on tightly, and put the bottles in the refrigerator. Avoid exposing the bottles to direct sunlight.[1]

** Please note that the above recipe should not be consumed without the approval of a medical doctor.

CHAPTER 16 Albarin: The Incredible, Injectable Cancer Cure

If you want my opinion, friends, aloe vera is one of the most impressive herbs out there today. Although it originally comes from East and South Africa, the earliest known references for the medicinal use of aloe comes from the ancient Egyptians who used it as a treatment for cuts, burns, and skin irritations. Beginning in the 1930s, aloe was used frequently for the treatment of minor skin ailments and for skin reactions from radiation burns.[1] But this single plant also offers amazing relief for constipation, psoriasis, frostbite, ulcerative colitis, and diabetes, too.

There are all sorts of studies on the uses of aloe, but more recent ones suggest that some components of aloe may also have anti-cancer effects by inhibiting an increase in cell numbers and inducing apoptosis (cell suicide) in human cancer cell lines. Along with its antioxidant and anti-inflammatory properties, that's a pretty impressive portfolio.

It was the amazing anti-cancer and immune boosting properties that inspired nutritionist Joe DiStephano and his partner, osteopath Dr. Daniel Mayer, to use aloe in their practice. They used an injectable form of aloe to treat the many cancer patients that came to them after all other treatments had failed—and it worked with great success. Many patients with no hope left were being given another chance to live with their injectable aloe formula, called Albarin.

But one day in 2002, tipped off by local oncologists who felt the Albarin was a threat to their livelihood, the FDA tried to put an end to the healing—and succeeded. Though this incredible treatment is no longer available in the U.S., fortunately there are other aloe products out there that offer similar effects, and like Albarin, may help keep cancer at bay.(2)

Kicking Your Immunity into High Gear

Recent studies suggest that some of the components of aloe, such as acemannan and aloeride may have immune-modulating (balancing to the immune system) and anti-cancer effects. Aloe is thought to have antioxidant and anti-inflammatory properties(2) and in addition, aloe vera has been shown to be effective against cancer in animals. In fact, in 1992, the U.S. Department of Agriculture actually approved the use of aloe vera for the treatment of soft tissue cancer in animals as well as feline leukemia.

Aloe also helps to lower the damage done to the body by treatments such as radiation and chemotherapy, which destroy healthy immune system cells that are very important for the body's recovery. With the use of aloe vera, the immune system gets a boost, tumors shrink, and metastases are reduced so the cancer does not spread.(3)

Some opponents of aloe claim that too much can be toxic. But in 1997 a study was conducted at the University of San Antonio to observe any negative effects of daily aloe consumption. Rather than exhibiting negative effects, test animals receiving daily aloe showed a remarkable reduction in leukemia, heart disease, and kidney disease. They concluded that there was no indication of harm done to the rats—even at high levels. The aloe-drinking animals actually lived 25 *percent longer* than those in the control group.(3)

Yet another study published in 1995 showed that aloe vera compounds called polysaccharides exhibited potent macrophage-activating capability, including producing increased volumes of nitric oxide (which has antitumor potential). And the list goes on and on.(4)

The Father of Aloe Vera and the FDA Raid

Ivan E. Danhof, Ph.D., M.D. is known as the world's leading expert on aloe vera and has over 30 years of laboratory research and extensive practical experience. Dr. Danhof has become recognized as one of the world's foremost experts on medically active herbal molecules, especially the functional components in aloe vera. After more than 20 years of research, Danhof developed the intravenous aloe vera preparation called Albarin. Not only has Dr. Danhoff published more than 80 research papers and served as a consultant to several pharmaceutical research institutes, he has also been a consultant to the FDA, serving on review panels and committees dealing primarily with gastrointestinal drugs.

Nutritionist Joe Di Stefano and osteopath Dr. Daniel Mayer had been using Albarin in their practice and observed that it appeared to be prolonging survival time of cancer patients in their clinic. Their use of Albarin with their clinic patients was also part of a program that was integral to the investigational new drug (IND) application for the Albarin treatment that Dr. Danhof had submitted to the FDA. DiStefano and Mayer observed that Albarin was causing tumor shrinkage, significant pain relief and increased energy levels and that advanced patients were achieving remission at an incredible rate of up to 94 percent.

But all was about to change.

In October of 2001, Joe Di Stefano exited his clinic at midnight after a long day and caught two strangers with rubber gloves on, sifting through his garbage dumpster and trespassing on his property without a search warrant. It turned out that these were FDA agents seeking evidence to obtain a search warrant against Joe Di Stefano's clinic. One week later, 120 agents from the FDA, DEA, Customs, U.S. Marshall's Service, Florida Department of Law Enforcement, and the Hillsborough County Sheriff's Office raided the Tampa and St. Petersburg clinics of Joe DiStefano and Dr. Mayer as well as Joe DiStefano's home. They warned the patients being treated at the clinic that it would be their last treatment with Albarin.

Alternatives to Albarin

Since the raids on the Florida clinics of DiStefano and Mayer, Albarin is no longer available for use in the U.S. Although it is a terrible shame that we don't have Albarin, fortunately there are other non-IV, aloe-based treatments available that are designed based on the research of Dr. Danhof and with principles similar to the Albarin. I've listed a few of these products here:

Aloe Vera Acemannan: Aloe Vera Acemannan is extracted from the species of aloe shown to have one of the highest levels of polymannan content (polymannans are the premium aloe nutrients). You can learn more about it at www.altcancer.com.

Serovera: This product contains the same "Aloe Mucilaginous Polysaccharides" that Albarin did. Each capsule contains 375mg of AMP extracted and freeze-dried under a controlled environment. To learn more about it, call (877)737-6267.[7]

CHAPTER 17

Cancer Treatment's New Frontier: Gene-Targeted Therapy

I've brought you some fascinating research on potential cancer cures from all corners of the world, but one of the most promising alternative treatments by far comes from a doctor in Houston, Texas. It's called Antineoplaston therapy and although it sounds more like something out of a science fiction novel, this breakthrough actually works together with the body's inborn biochemical defense system to convert cancerous cells back to normal functioning.

Since his amazing discovery, Dr. Stanislaw Burzynski has been treating cancer patients successfully in his Houston clinic for the past 30 years—with no help from the FDA or Big Pharma. In fact, they've both spent the last 30 years trying to stymie the approval of this incredible treatment. Despite the many roadblocks he's encountered along the way, Dr. Burzynski's safe and non-toxic treatment for cancer is available and giving new hope to cancer patients everywhere.

"The Body Itself Has the Treatment for Cancer"

Antineoplastons are actually short chains of amino acids or protein building blocks called peptides, derived from two or more amino acids. According to Dr. Burzynski, these peptides act as molecular switches, which turn off the life processes in cancer cells and force them to die through programmed cell death—or commit cell suicide.

Unlike chemo and radiation, which destroy all of your cells—good and bad— Antineoplastons work to target cancer cells only and leave your healthy cells alone.

"Obviously what we know about cancer today is quite different than what we knew several years ago," says Dr. Burzynski. "From the very beginning I theorized that they turn on the genes that fight cancer, known as tumor-suppressor genes, and turn off oncogenes, so this was...when I realized that cancer is a genetic disease."

Dr. Burzynski later found that Antineoplastons could be divided into two groups: those with broad-spectrum activity against cancer, and those with effects against certain types of cancer.[2]

FDA Roadblocks

While Dr. Burzynski's incredible Antineoplaston discovery was made over 30 years ago, clinical trials on the therapy only began in 1995, and it comes as no surprise that the FDA and Big Pharma played a big part in slowing down recognition and approval over the years. In fact, Dr. Burzynski himself shared the following:

> *"They did whatever they could to slow me down and tried to put me to prison for life, and one of the reasons was...some of the people making decisions about our treatment were working for the pharmaceutical companies which were trying to steal what*

we had. The government, together with pharmaceutical companies, was simply trying to steal my patents...and there is no secret about it. The guys from the FDA who did a lot of wrong things are no longer working at the FDA. The pharmaceutical company trying to steal my invention and patents went bankrupt and some of the insurance companies...also had problems. So we did quite well in an extremely difficult circumstance."[2]

Dr. Burzynski even encountered resistance from fellow medical doctors who were threatened by his discovery. Though some congratulated him on his work, others "reported me to the Texas Medical Board, saying that I was using medicine that was not advised for this type of cancer, even though the patient responded greatly to the treatment. [In] every way I encountered a lot of resistance...Finally I was sued and filed a lawsuit against the United States and won...I still encounter a lot of resistance from the Government [but] they are forced to work with me under the pressure of public opinion."

In spite of the FDA's resistance and the threats of certain pharmaceutical companies, today Dr. Burzynski's clinic is the site of FDA-run clinical trials which have already reached Stage 3, the final step before government approval in the United States. In fact, four of the Antineoplaston-based medicines created by Dr. Burzynski are in the final stages of the approval process and two are already approved for use in other medical conditions and are available as prescription medications in the U.S. under the names phenylbutyrate and phenylacetate.[3]

A Personalized Approach: Get Treated for YOUR Cancer

According to Dr. Burzynski, the goal of cancer treatment is to treat the disease that has resulted from changes in your genes during everyday life. How do they treat those changes? By disrupting a network of about a hundred genes (out of approximately 2,400) which are involved in a typical cancer case. This, in a nutshell, is the function of Antineoplastons and the personalized therapy being used at the Burzynski Clinic today.

Right now, full Antineoplaston therapy is only available by IV to patients who qualify to enter one of the FDA clinical trials being conducted on the therapy. As of this book's publication, there are 17 open clinical trials on Antineoplastons, encompassing a wide range of cancer types in both children and adults and all are being supervised and monitored by the FDA.[3]

If you don't qualify to enter a clinical trial, you still have the option to receive personalized treatment, which includes Antineoplaston therapy administered as phenylbutyrate and phenylacetate in oral tablet form, combined with one or more gene-targeted medications which work on between 2-14 genes. You'll get specific testing to determine which medications is the best match for you. This combination, plus the proper supplements and diet, provides you with broad-spectrum coverage. Then, adding two or three other powerful medications knocks out and speeds up tumor elimination.

This sort of personalized approach is almost unheard of in conventional cancer treatments where doctors pretty much treat your cancer, not YOU—and treat every cancer of a certain type in the same way. Not to mention the fact that Antineoplastons have very manageable side effects, if any (some people feel a bit thirstier and some get a rash—no comparison to the side effects from chemo and radiation!).

According to Dr. Burzynski, "gene-targeted therapeutics selected based on genetic testing and used in combination yield total results from the synergistic activity of all medications. The indiscriminate use of expensive gene-targeted therapeutics without identification of proper candidates for treatments costs numerous human lives and billions of dollars spent on useless medications, which could help other patients who are good candidates."

In other words, the proper medications for disrupting cancer genes already exist if oncologists would just learn to use them properly.

Of the two forms of treatment (oral and IV), Dr. Burzynski prefers to administer Antineoplastons intravenously along with gene-targeted therapy, but, with the state of affairs today, he lamented that "unfortunately this is a weird period of time when we have more like totalitarian medicine, so the way I see the patients is more or less dictated by the bureaucrats."[2] So, most often, the oral approach is used.

Good Nutrition to Fit Your Genes

Today, the Burzynski Clinic offers alternative cancer treatments for over 50 different types of cancer, including colon, pulmonary, breast, prostate, head and neck, ovarian, pancreatic, esophageal, hepatic, renal, bladder, brain, malignant melanoma, lymphoma, and many others. In addition to Antineoplastons and gene-targeted medications, the Burzynski Clinic has dietary specialists on staff to recommend specific diets according to your individual genetic needs.

The Burzynski team also recommends taking supplements like curcumin (see Chapter 9) that help keep tumor suppressor genes functioning normally. Dr. Burzynski believes that "in the future, [diet and supplements] should be personalized too...begin[ning] with screening of genetic activity in a particular patient and then designing the proper plan for that patient...our task will be to impede these genes with diet and proper supplements before the cancer will happen."

Are Antineoplastons THE Cure for Cancer?

As I've told you before, labeling anything a cure for all cancer is a near-impossible feat since the term, "cancer" is an umbrella which holds beneath it many different types of diseases. But, for many patients, Antineoplaston and personalized therapy may hold the key to a full recovery.

Some of the best success seen with Antineoplastons have been in the most common type of brain tumor in children, astrocytomas, where the failure rate is only 7 percent. That means 93 percent of patients with this type of tumor respond well to Antineoplaston therapy. And between 60 and 70 percent of these patients will either get rid of their tumors completely or—at the very least—have them shrink by more than 50 percent.

There is also a 60 percent response rate with breast cancer. And with prostate cancer, the success rate is a whopping 91 percent. These are incredible stats but remember, it's important to keep in mind that they can give you only approximate information, since every patient must be treated individually.

The Future of Cancer Treatment

Antineoplaston therapy has been around for over 30 years, and, aside from the mountain of scientific evidence in its favor, there are hundreds and hundreds of real people who are alive and well today, here to tell their success and recovery stories thanks to Dr. Burzynski's brilliant discovery. Antineoplastons are celebrated today by "people who have been cancer-free for 10, 20 and 30 years...We still have patients whom we cannot help, but a good number of patients can get rid of their cancer and this can be done now."

Amazingly, Dr. Burzynski has been able to work within the system despite the impossible odds that were once against him, and FDA approval is just a step away. Since a big part of the future of cancer treatment is on the genetic level, Antineoplastons are definitely ahead of the game and may one day leave traditional therapies like chemo and radiation by the wayside.

According to Dr. Burzynski, the conventional treatments for cancer are "archaic" and "since radiation is over one hundred years of age [invented] when the knowledge of cancer was at its infancy [and] chemo was introduced over 60 years ago...we can compare it to the middle ages of medicine and they will [both] disappear in the next 10 years or so."

If the amazing results he's achieved with Antineoplaston therapy are any indication, he could very well be right.

If you're interested in receiving Antineoplaston therapy or Dr. Burzynski's personalized cancer therapy, contact the info-line at the Burzynski Clinic by calling (800)714-7181. A cancer information specialist will help to assess whether the treatment is right for you and how you should proceed. For general information, visit www.burzynskiclinic.com.

There are also two great books about Dr. Burzynski and Antineoplaston therapy you may want to consider reading: *Galileo's Lawyer* by Richard A. Jaffe and *The Burzynski Breakthrough* by Thomas D. Elias.

CHAPTER 18 The Herbal Salve that Saved an Astronaut

"There are people in this world—and I'm one of them—who know that most cancers pose a medical challenge no greater than curing athlete's foot. The official establishment's success in sustaining the Great Cancer Ruse as a leading cash cow has killed untold tens of millions of people. It presents a medical, social, political, and economic scandal of the highest magnitude—one for which I challenge anyone to find an equal."

—Greg Caton, herbalist and formulator of Cansema

Do you believe in synchronicity?

You know, the things in life that seem to have no relation at all, but end up being meaningful in a truly extraordinary way? If not, what you're about to read will undoubtedly change your mind. the story of herbalist Greg Caton, his product, Cansema, *and* that of scientist and former United States astronaut, Dr. Brian O'Leary, who recently experienced an extraordinary recovery from skin cancer by using it.

According to Dr. Brian O'Leary, he has recently joined the ranks of those that have been successfully treated with Cansema, a formula with a 100-year history of curing skin cancer. But, again, despite its efficacy, Cansema and its creator, Greg Caton, have long been subject to a world of harassment and suppression, emphasizing for us what we've learned to be true time and time again: When a formula can't be patented, no drug company will even look in its direction. Actually, the very existence of Cansema is such a powerful threat to the cancer industry that they've tried nearly everything in their power to stop its use, including an overwhelming attempt to destroy the life of the man who formulated it.

But before we get into that, let's go back to the story of Dr. Brian O'Leary.

Sidestepping Surgery

Dr. O'Leary had been suffering with an incurable lesion on his back for three years, and the pain was getting progressively worse over time. Left with no choice but to schedule a biopsy, he was told by doctors that his lesion was actually basal cell carcinoma—and it would have to be removed.

"I've had surgery before in my life and I know it's not very pleasant," he said. "Doctors usually underestimate the side effects of surgery and...it was only with great reluctance that I agreed to it."

Just three days before he was due to go in for the operation that would remove a large portion of his back tissue, O'Leary got an unexpected visit from a friend of a friend. It was herbalist Greg Caton—who just happened to be the creator of an alternative skin cancer salve called Cansema. After a long conversation with Caton and some further research, Dr. O'Leary decided to go with his gut: He cancelled the surgery and tried the salve.

According to O'Leary, "...It seemed to selectively seek out the cancer cells and attack them. And although it took three applications over a period of about three months, now it's virtually all gone."

Amazingly spared from surgery and the potential for continuing years of pain, Dr. O'Leary feels immense gratitude for having had the option to use Cansema. "Right now," he said, "I'm feeling pretty good and quite healed! The thing on my back is...nothing like it was before I started taking the Cansema...this treatment worked so well that I didn't have to have surgery... so that's basically my... very happy story."(1)

Cansema's Long Healing History

So what, you ask, is this incredible formula and where on Earth did it come from? Well, Cansema has quite a story in its own right, one that started back in the 16th century with Paracelsus, who used a formula made of "sal ammoniac" (ammonium chloride), along with fuligo (wood soot), and orpiment (arsenic sulfide) to treat skin cancers and wounds.(2)

Later, in the mid-19th century when Native American herbs became very popular in Europe, Dr. J.W. Fell, from the Middlesex Hospital in London, developed a paste made of bloodroot, zinc chloride, flour, and water which he found, if applied to a malignant growth, generally destroyed the tumor within two to four weeks.(3)

The late Dr. Raymond Christopher also created and used a similar ointment that contained potent anti-cancer herbs such as poke root and black walnut bark, which was used to draw out cancers and tumors from the skin.

These original skin-cancer salve formulas all contain a compound called zinc chloride, plus one or more medicinal herbs with anti-microbial properties, like bloodroot, bittersweet, ginger root, galanga, and even capsicum (from cayenne pepper), which puts them into a category called escharotics. Though the root of the word "escharotic" means "burning," (the word is usually used in conventional medicine to describe the effects of a skin burn caused by acid or other chemicals) no actual burning occurs with Cansema use. In fact, this formula has the incredible ability to differentiate between cancerous cells and healthy cells, and seeks out and destroys the cancer while leaving healthy tissue alone. And within less than two months, the cancer disappears.[4]

Caton, Cansema, and the FDA Clash

Greg Caton had years of involvement in the alternative medicine business along with a particular passion for unique herbal formulas, but it was only in 1990 that his life changed in one moment that he, like O'Leary, feels was synchronicity.

One day, while going about his business, he was approached by a fellow businessman who had heard about a zinc chloride and blood-

The Sum of Its Parts

Bloodroot (Sanguinarea canadensis) is an eastern North American woodland herb that was commonly used to treat cancer by Native Americans. It is as a primary ingredient in most escharotic salves and pastes and has been found to possess powerful anti-cancer properties.

The more controversial ingredient in Cansema is zinc chloride. Although it can cause serious burns if applied in high concentrations, the quantities of zinc chloride in Cansema are too small to cause such damage. In fact, Cansema is very selective in its action: It is lethal for cancerous tissue and only mildly irritating to healthy skin.[3]

root formula that cured cancer from another complete stranger who he'd struck up a random conversation with at a gas station.

Though there was seemingly no relation at the time, it was an

How it Works

There are six steps involved in Cansema treatment. Fair warning to those of you who are squeamish—they are a bit graphic.

1. **Eschar formation:** After application of Cansema, the cancerous lesion forms into a scab, or "eschar." The cancer is completely dead, but the healing process has only begun.
2. **Edema & isolation:** There is a buildup of antibodies and blood serum in the surrounding tissue, which causes a reddening and general puffiness (but this varies from case to case). The eschar becomes better defined from the surrounding, healthy, non-cancerous tissue.
3. **Eschar containment:** The eschar begins to dry up like a scab. As healthy skin is formed underneath the eschar, it is slowly ejected from the body and the redness disappears.
4. **Eschar expulsion:** The entire eschar gets ejected naturally by the body when the last connective skin tissue beneath it is broken or deteriorates.
5. **Decavitation:** A pit-like area remains where the tumor was ejected. Since the skin layers have not completely formed, the area can look extremely raw and unprotected. Vitamin E or petroleum jelly is applied to minimize scarring and aid the healing process.
6. **Final healing:** The epidermal layers re-grow and usually there is minimal scarring and discoloration.

event that, similar to his future meeting with Dr. O'Leary, would become meaningful in an extraordinary way. Indeed, shortly thereafter, Caton and his wife started a supplement company called Alpha Omega Labs which, among other products, manufactured the very escharotic formula the businessman had mentioned to him previously. And over the next 10+ years, Cansema helped cure thousands of cancer cases.[2]

It's rare that a product with such incredible success goes unnoticed for too long by the FDA—and in the case of Cansema, the FDA not only took notice, but they also used two previous civil lawsuits that had been filed against Alpha Omega Labs as justification to raid Caton's home and arrest him.

But according to Caton, even without the two lawsuits, Cansema never stood a chance to be approved for use as a cancer treatment by the FDA, a status which can only be obtained if a pharmaceutical company submits a new drug application and successfully completes a process that costs hundreds of millions of dollars.

As he sees it, "modern medicine is built around the phony concept…that the things that are most curative are in instances where you can point to a singular molecular entity that does the job. We know as herbalists that there are combinations of chemicals and subtle energies that work in synergistic fashions to produce the desired results...so whether we did or did not make a claim [to cure cancer] with Cansema it would never, never, never get approval."

Freedom to Heal

Today, Greg Caton lives in Ecuador and works with practitioners who treat advanced cancer patients with proven alternative techniques. Under Article 44 of Ecuador's Constitution, citizens have broad latitude to choose the systems of health care they want—freedoms that Americans can only dream of.

The Cases Against Cansema

The first civil case against Greg Caton involved a woman from Texas who claimed that she had been burned by an Alpha Omega Labs product called H3O that her surgeon had used on her to speed up the wound healing process during post-op. According to Caton, the product didn't possess the properties necessary to inflict the injury, and when Caton's insurance company refused to pay the woman, she went right to the FDA for help. And help she got. She received a total of *$500,000* from insurance companies representing Caton, the surgeon, and the hospital.[2]

In the second case, a nurse in Indiana sued Alpha Omega Labs claiming that *either* Cansema or another product "took (her) nose off," although she **also** testified that one or the other product cured her cancer. Still—the insurance company settled the case for $800,000 as a result of the FDA's criminal charges against Caton.

Needless to say, these cases initially caused a media frenzy, and shortly afterwards, Caton got a knock on the door from FBI agents, who arrested him and charged him for a completely unrelated "crime" (firearms possession—including an heirloom shotgun that his wife's grandfather had passed down to her—something which clearly had nothing to do with the cases). Eight months later, the charge was dropped and replaced with FDA charges, primarily based "on this nurse who said that her nose got burned off by using a product we sold called H3O."

Two months later, the FDA's victim stated in her sworn deposition that she never even applied the H3O, and that she originally purchased it with the intent to try to win money from a lawsuit!

The Legality of Cansema

In most countries of the world, Cansema is completely legal as a cancer remedy, but in most Western countries one cannot technically say what it does or what it's for (i.e., make a "claim") because of the Dietary Supplement Health and Education Act of 1994, or DSHEA.

So, although Cansema is an effective topical skin cancer salve, Cansema is not an approved drug as defined by the U.S. Food & Drug Administration, or any of its European counterparts, therefore it's illegal for a company inside the U.S. to sell a product like Cansema as a cancer remedy, despite its history of effectiveness.

Caton explained that "in almost every…area of health care, the indigenous communities trust their own people more than they do outsiders…when a patient is ill, whether a high paid NY attorney or a simple *compesino* living in the jungle, they want relief…they want results."

Caton also believes strongly in the link between nutrition and cancer and recommends the approach of Dr. Max Gerson (see Chapter 7), along with a variety of different herbal remedies. He believes that the modern diets are substantially deficient in natural minerals, vitamins, essential oils, and "nutritional compounds and vital energies that modern science has not discovered, recognized or cannot even articulate."

Caton also recommends colon hydrotherapy, or high colonics, to most of his customers, believing that "no matter what you do to help a cancer patient, if they are wallowing in their own filth internally you're not going to help unless part of what you're doing is addressing these toxicity issues." He noted that "the modern diet is significantly depleted in fiber and…one of the casualties of the way we eat is that the colon tends to suffer as a result and is more likely to get impacted." He has found that this therapy is particularly important when the patient has already gone through conventional cancer treatments. "When the hospitals finish using chemo and radiation, we find that people's colons are in horrific states and need to be repaired and detoxified."[6]

Where to Find This Miracle Salve

I'm going to go out on a limb and guess that you don't live in Ecuador, and chances are, it's not your first choice for your next vacation. But that doesn't mean you can't get your hands on Cansema. Currently, there are four versions of the Cansema formula (the original, plus a penetrating "deep tissue," "iodine," and veterinary variation). Additionally, there are two internal variations of Cansema (the original Cansema Tonic I) and a formula without zinc (Cansema Tonic III). The company has since discontinued Cansema in capsule form.

Remember that although Cansema is designed for self-administration, this is no replacement for proper medical advice which I recommend you seek, as always. You should also keep in mind that the application of Cansema can produce some pain, so you may want to be sure you have some sort of painkiller readily available before beginning to use it.

For more information on Cansema, contact Alpha Omega Labs by calling (888)450-7909, or visit *www.herbhealers.com*.

Though Cansema has had a long and difficult journey—and there's still a long way to go—the persistence of people like Caton has paved the way for a future that will hopefully be a bit brighter for the world of cancer treatment.

CHAPTER 19 Nurse Caisse's Anti-Cancer Herbal Brew

"Tremendous sums have been raised and appropriated for official cancer research during the past 50 years, with almost nothing new or productive discovered. It would make these foundations look pretty silly, if an obscure Canadian nurse discovered an effective treatment for cancer!"

—Rene Caisse

One of the true originals in our eclectic collection of alternative cancer cures from around the world is an ancient Native American concoction that's been used for hundreds of years to fight cancer—and the story behind it is quite extraordinary.

I'm talking about Essiac tea, a blend of powerful herbs discovered by Canadian nurse Rene Caisse to be a potent weapon against cancer of all kinds. In her day, Nurse Caisse had such success with Essiac that she even came to be known as Canada's Cancer Nurse, treating thousands of patients who came from far and wide to receive treatment with her then-secret herbal formula.

Despite years of success in beating cancer, conventional medicine never gave its stamp of approval to Essiac's efficacy, and the Canadian government repeatedly attempted to halt its use. Nevertheless, the clinical evidence collected by Caisse and many others that has mounted over the years has clearly shown us the power of this synergistic herbal blend.

An Incredible Herbal Discovery

It all started back in 1922, when Canadian nurse, Rene Caisse noticed some scar tissue on the breast of an elderly woman in her care—the result of cancer that she had been diagnosed with years before. When asked about her scar, the elderly woman explained to her nurse that she shunned the idea of breast surgery and did not have the money for it anyway, and to her luck, shortly thereafter, she met an old Indian medicine man who told her that he could cure this same breast cancer with an herbal tea. She boldly decided to take his advice as well as his tea, and nearly 30 years later, she was alive and well enough to pass on the list of powerful herbs to Caisse.

The list sat on Caisse's desk until a year later, when during a leisurely garden stroll, a retired doctor friend told Caisse that if more people would use the herb sheep sorrel, "there would be little cancer in the world." Remembering the same common herb from the old medicine man's blend, Nurse Caisse decided she would test this herbal tea on herself if she ever developed cancer. But her opportunity came sooner than expected: Caisse's aunt developed stomach cancer and was given only six months to live by her doctors, who had nothing else to offer her in terms of treatment.

With nothing to lose, Caisse gave her aunt the herbal tea treatment with her doctor's consent—and the result? Her aunt lived for 21 more years, cancer-free.

Caisse later gave the tea to her own 72-year-old mother who

was diagnosed with inoperable cancer of the liver and given only days to live, and she too enjoyed life cancer-free for another 18 years after taking the herbal tea.[1]

The Essiac Formula

The original list given to Nurse Caisse by the elderly woman included eight different herbs and over the years, she was able to perfect a formula based on this list by testing various herbal combinations on lab mice and on human cancer patients. The original formula included: burdock root, slippery elm inner bark, sheep sorrel, Indian rhubarb root, watercress, blessed thistle, red clover, and kelp, but after much research, Caisse was able to reduce her tea to four main herbs that she found to be the most effective for treating cancer: burdock root, sheep sorrel, slippery elm and Indian rhubarb. She named her formula Essiac—or Caisse spelled backwards.

Soon thereafter, Nurse Caisse opened and ran a cancer clinic under the supervision and observation of a number of doctors, and treated thousands of patients with her secret Essiac formula. She and the doctors worked hard to discover which herb was most effective in reducing tumors, by administering injections of each of the separate herbs. When they pinpointed the tumor-reducing herb, they gave it to patients by injection and the three others were given to patients as a tea to detoxify the body.

Nurse Caisse treated thousands of cancer patients with Essiac, *free of charge,* and her treatments were so effective that in 1938, 55,000 signatures were compiled for a petition presented to the Ontario legislature to authorize her to practice medicine in Ontario in the treatment of cancer. The bill failed to pass by just three votes and that same year, Canadian medical authorities investigated her clinic, promptly pronouncing Essiac "ineffective."[1] Apparently, control of the medical system by influential "powers-that-be" isn't restricted to just the United States!

Pressure from the Medical Establishment

Caisse herself was not initially aware at the time of the control that the medical and pharmaceutical establishment possessed, stating herself that "I did not know then of an organized effort to keep a cancer cure from being discovered, especially by an independent researcher not affiliated with any organization supported by private or public funds." For us, it comes as no surprise that the medical establishment was such a threat to Caisse, since Essiac is cheap and non-toxic. And the fact that she took no money for her treatments didn't help things. In fact, it meant that her very existence was in direct opposition to the medical establishment, which focused almost solely on the lucrative profits to be made from cancer treatment.

After the petition was delivered to the National Health and Welfare Department in Ontario, she began to experience continuous threats of arrest until she finally chose to withdraw from the public eye.

Ultimately, Nurse Caisse was forced to close her clinic in 1942 and, exhausted by the constant investigations, she brought her four-herb formula to Dr. Charles Brusch's clinic. They became partners and shortly thereafter, they returned to the original eight-herb blend, which they gave as an herbal tea, just as the Ojibwa Indians had originally.

In 1977, Caisse finally gave her secret four-herb formula over to the Resperin Corporation of Ontario, just one year before her death, with the intent of having it tested and sold. Caisse sold her Essiac formula for a symbolic one dollar, finally feeling she had found a company that could help fulfill her promise of healing to mankind.

But only a few years after her death, in 1982, Resperin's studies on Essiac were shut down by the Canadian government once again, with claims that their research methods were "flawed."

The Proof Behind the Promise

Each of the herbs in Essiac has its own chemical make-up and effect on the body, and there are plenty of studies out there on the unique functions:

Burdock root: In 1966, Hungarian researchers discovered anti-tumor activity in Burdock Root due to inulin, which attaches to white blood cells and enhances their function.[3] It also contains benzaldehyde, which has significant anti-cancer effects in humans.

Sheep sorrel: A staple of folk medicine, Sheep Sorrel was used in cancer treatment as early as the 1740's. It is rich in vitamins and minerals, and contains chlorophyll, which helps to carry oxygen

Essiac's Recipe for Success

Rene Caisse spent her life refining the formula with her hands-on research, a tedious job since every herbal formula has its own synergy and creates a specific effect, which can change with the alteration of just one ingredient in the formula. The recipe below was the final formula created after decades of experimentation and research with real cancer patients:

- 6 ½ cups of burdock root
- 1 pound of sheep sorrel, powdered
- ¼ pound of slippery elm bark, powdered
- 1 ounce of Turkish rhubarb root, powdered

Mix ingredients well and store in glass jar in dark dry cupboard. Use 1 ounce of herb mixture to 32 ounces of water. Boil rapidly for 10 minutes (covered) then turn off heat and leave on warm plate over night (covered). In the morning, heat until steaming hot and let settle a few minutes, then strain through fine strainer into hot sterilized bottles and let cool. Store in a dark cool cupboard. The tea must be refrigerated after opening.[2]

to the cells of the body. As a folk remedy, it has also been used to relieve bruises and burns.

Slippery elm: It has been shown to possess anti-tumor activity and is an anti-inflammatory for the digestive system. It also lubricates bones and joints, and contains fatty acids. Fatty acids similar to those in slippery elm have been shown to boost the immune system in studies on mice.[4]

Indian rhubarb root: Rich in iron, Indian rhubarb helps to purge the liver and the rest of the body of wastes. Like sheep sorrel, it contains aloe emodin, which have been shown to inhibit tumors in animal tests.[5,6]

Though there are plenty of studies out there on the individual herbs, few trials have been carried out on Essiac as a whole.

Dr. Brusch conducted a few experiments at his medical center near Boston and one study on mice injected with human cancer cells showed that Essiac killed tumors at a higher rate than seen in control mice. Dr. Brusch even successfully used Essiac in his own battle with bowel cancer. He also wrote in a notarized letter that Essiac "reduces pain and causes a recession in [tumor] growth. Patients gained weight and showed a great improvement in their general health...In some cases, if the tumor didn't disappear, it could be surgically removed after Essiac with less risk of metastasis."

A more recently published in vitro study on Essiac, conducted in 2004, on prostate cancer cells showed that at low doses Essiac may be able to inhibit tumor cell growth while enhancing immune response.[8] In addition, in 2006, two studies, both conducted in Toronto, were presented at a meeting of naturopathic physicians. The first showed increased cytotoxicity toward prostate cancer cells as well as significant antioxidant properties.[9] The second, in which Essiac was administered to rats, demonstrated Essiac's positive gastric protection.[10]

I've seen the effects of Essiac first hand: Early in my practice, a father brought his 13-year-old son in to see me because the boy had developed a firm, ugly mass on his knee. I urged the father to have it diagnosed, and when he did, it came back as cancer so bad that it would require *experimental* chemotherapy. The doctors told him he had no choice, that he had to go through this dangerous treatment, and that the boy would most likely lose the leg above the knee anyway. The father refused and then found out he would be turned in for child abuse (yes, child abuse) for refusing medical "standard-of-care."

Experimental chemotherapy as standard care? That's a good one.

So this man did what any other father would do when the life of his child is at stake. He fought for his son's life by fleeing to Canada in the middle of the night. And that was the last I thought I'd hear from the family. Then, about three years later, a lanky teenager walked into my office. It was that same boy, no lump on his knee, both legs working just fine. The father followed behind, saying they couldn't stay, because there was still an outstanding warrant for his arrest. But he had wanted me to see how Essiac had cured his son.

Finding the Real Deal

There are many versions of Essiac tea out there today, which can be confusing when you're searching for the best quality formula and product. In fact, I can understand why Rene Caisse kept her four-herb Essiac formula a secret: She didn't trust people to make it properly and thought that it would be altered.

Dr. Brusch signed over the rights to the eight-herb Essiac formula in 1988 which ultimately resulted in the world-wide manufacturing and distribution rights being passed onto Flora Inc. in 1992. Today, their Essiac product is known as FlorEssence. Meanwhile, Resperin, the company that received the four-herb formula directly from Rene Caisse, has since gone out of business, but not before transferring the rights to the Essiac formula to Essiac Canada International.

They offer both the original powdered combination of herbs, as well as a more convenient liquid version. So, technically there are two legitimate formulas on the marketplace today—Essiac as manufactured by Essiac Canada International, and FlorEssence as manufactured by Flora. If I were to use Essiac as part of a treatment program for cancer, I'd definitely go for one of the aforementioned products and avoid the other versions that are out there, which are actually deviations from the two original Essiac formulas.[11] Contact information for the two companies is listed below.

Although there's a lot of evidence in its favor, I must emphasize that Essiac tea is probably best used as an addition to other cancer protocols, not as a main treatment. Do check with your doctor first to see if the following applies for you, but generally Essiac can safely be taken in conjunction with other cancer treatments, and can be taken every day. In addition to being used for cancer treatment, Essiac can be used preventatively to keep your immune system healthy.

If you do decide to try Essiac, I would follow in Rene Caisse's footsteps and drink your tea within 48 hours of making it. If ordered by mail, it may be several months old or even older, if you consider how long it might have taken to get to you after having been dehydrated, processed and stored. Obviously, if you can grow your own herbs, that's best. But remember, as always, whatever you decide to add to your cancer protocol, do check with your doctor first!

Essiac Canada International
(888)-900-2299
www.essiac-canada-intl.com

Flora Inc. USA
(800)446-2110
www.florahealth.com

CHAPTER 20

The Cancer-Killing Supervitamin

You've probably been guzzling it down in your tall glass of OJ every morning for years and popping pills of it each day to prevent the common cold. Yes friends, I'm referring to good old-fashioned vitamin C. We've known for years that it's a key antioxidant, critical for preventing chronic disease, but believe it or not, vitamin C plays an integral role in the treatment of cancer as well.

Back in the 1970s, it was American biochemist Linus Pauling who discovered that one of the most inexpensive and commonly used nutrients around also has the ability to act as a potent, natural form of chemotherapy when given intravenously. Shortly after his discovery, however, the possibility of treatment with IV vitamin C quickly became clouded over with controversy, and the poor research methods used in the clinical studies only served to kick it further to the wayside.

The good news is that scientists have once again begun to re-examine the value of IV vitamin C as a treatment for cancer—and the results thus far are looking more than promising in clinics all over the country.

The Little Vitamin with Big Potential

In order to understand how vitamin C can reverse some cancers, I'm going to back up a bit and explain how it does its job in our bodies...

On a day-to-day basis, vitamin C helps to form collagen, an important protein used to your make skin, tendons, ligaments, and blood vessels, and it's essential for the healing of wounds and the repair of bones and teeth. Since vitamin C is water soluble (meaning your body can't store it and any excess that's present in your blood is expelled though urine), you need a constant and continuous supply of it in your diet to meet your body's needs at any given time.

You may have also heard vitamin C called an antioxidant, or a nutrient that blocks free radical damage. Just to remind you, free radicals are by-products of everyday living and breathing, but are produced much more during exercise and exposure to smoke and chemicals. Their accumulation is largely responsible for aging and the development of all kinds of health conditions.

But one of the lesser known and most important roles of vitamin C is to defend us against tumor growth. Vitamin C is required for our immune systems to generate and mobilize the specialized cells that fight cancer and infections. The problem is, the more stress your immune system is under, the more of your vitamin C is used up.

To sum it up, vitamin C has many important roles and since your body doesn't make it and can't store it long term, you need to take in lots of it. But just how much you need and how you should take it have long been at the center of the vitamin C-cancer debate.[1]

5 Fast Facts about Vitamin C

- Vitamin C is critical for life
- Most mammals make their own vitamin C internally—human beings are one of the very rare exceptions
- Over-cooking destroys vitamin C in foods
- The adult RDA for vitamin C is 90 mg a day for men and 75 for women

The Cancer-Killing Vitamin

In 1966, Dr. Ewan Cameron pointed out that the "intercellular cement" that binds the cells of normal tissues can be broken down by tumor-produced enzymes. A few years later, in 1973, Dr. Cameron, together with Linus Pauling, PhD, popularized the notion that vitamin C could stimulate normal cells to inhibit these enzymes.

Soon afterwards, Drs. Pauling and Cameron began to conduct a number of studies to test the efficacy of vitamin C in cancer patients. In their 1976 study, 100 subjects with terminal cancer were given supplemental vitamin C (10 grams/daily) intravenously and compared to a control group of 1,000 patients of similar status treated by the same clinicians in the same Scotland hospital. They found that the average survival time was more than 4.2 times greater for the patients given IV vitamin C than it was for the controls.

By August 1976 (five years after the beginning of the study) 18 of the 100 vitamin C-treated patients were still living while all of the controls had died. Overall, the 100 ascorbic acid-treated patients lived, on the average, 300 days longer than their matched controls with better quality of life.[2]

A second study performed in 1978 with 100 new ascorbic acid-treated patients and 1,000 controls broke down the improved patient survival times by cancer type. The researchers found that for each type of cancer, there was an improvement in survival.[3]

Research Roadblock

As we already know, mainstream medicine doesn't accept such concepts as vitamins providing a viable treatment for cancer so quickly. So it shouldn't come as much of a surprise that when researchers at the Mayo Clinic tested Pauling and Cameron's findings in two of their own randomized placebo-controlled studies in 1979, they found no differences in outcome between terminal cancer patients receiving 10 grams of vitamin C per day versus those given a placebo.

How is it that such a drastic difference in results occurred between Pauling and Cameron's studies and those done at the Mayo Clinic?

The most obvious reason is that Pauling and Cameron administered the vitamin C by IV and the Mayo Clinic study gave it orally, a difference that Pauling knew then and we know today to be a crucial one in terms of vitamin C's bioavailability and effect. After all, intravenous (IV) administration can result in much higher blood levels than oral administration. And levels that are toxic to certain types of cancer cells in culture can be achieved only with intravenous administration of vitamin C.[4]

Recently, two well-respected researchers from the National Institutes of Health (NIH) suggested that the route of administration may have indeed been the key to the discrepancy found in the 1970s. In their 2004 study, 17 healthy hospitalized volunteers were given either oral or intravenous doses of vitamin C, and blood plasma levels were calculated for a dose range of 1 to 100 grams. They found that "peak plasma vitamin C concentrations were higher after administration of intravenous doses than after administration of oral doses." In fact, the blood concentration of vitamin C when given intravenously was 6.6 times greater than when the same amount was given orally.[5]

The Key to C

With these incredible results on the table, the natural question that arises is: What the heck is IV vitamin C actually doing to fight cancer so well? Well, the exact mechanism is still unknown—but we know that part of the story is that it causes the accelerated pro-oxidant damage of tumor cells.

To put it simply, when the absorption of vitamin C is increased and the levels go up so much, it starts to act as a pro-oxidant instead of antioxidant, as I mentioned earlier, because it starts to interact with the copper and iron in our cells, causing a reaction which produces small amounts of hydrogen peroxide, (the same peroxide that you apply to cuts and scrapes to kill germs). Interestingly, human white blood cells are able to make and break down their own peroxide to kill germs, which cancer cells are not able to do because they lack the enzyme catalase. Bottom line: the high-dose IV vitamin C produces peroxide, and continued build-up of peroxide makes the cancer cell burst.[6]

I must mention here that many conventional oncologists will tell you that small doses of vitamin C may actually help cancer cells by allowing them to arm themselves against the free-radical induced damage caused by chemotherapy and radiation. But remember: only markedly higher doses of vitamin C will selectively build up as peroxide in the cancer cells to the point of killing them, and these tumor-toxic dosages can only be obtained by intravenous administration.[7]

The Future of IV Vitamin C

Though it's been around for decades and was once brushed aside by the conventional medical community, IV vitamin C is definitely making a comeback. New research and evidence for the efficacy of IV vitamin C as an anti-cancer treatment is emerging, slowly but surely, and the word is being spread far and wide about this incredible alternative cancer treatment.

In 2006, the *Canadian Medical Association Journal* published the details of three IV C/cancer case studies which show us first-hand, the power of this incredible vitamin.[8]

Case One: A 51-year-old woman with kidney tumors refused conventional treatment and instead, received 65 grams of IVC twice each week in addition to other. After 10 months of IVC, her tumors were gone and her cancer remained in complete remission for four years.

Case Two: A 49-year-old man with a bladder tumor and multiple satellite tumors, declined chemotherapy and radiation and instead began an IVC regimen of 30 grams twice each week for three months, followed by 30 grams once every two months for four years. During those four years he sometimes took more frequent treatments. Nine years later, the man is in good health with no recurrence or spreading of the cancer. The authors of the CMAJ article note that standard treatment for muscle invasive bladder cancer is complete or partial bladder removal. When treated without surgery, this cancer type "almost invariably" spreads to other organs "within a short period."

Case Three: After six weeks of radiation therapy to treat lymphoma, a 66-year-old woman declined chemotherapy and began receiving 15 grams of IVC twice each week for two months. She continued with a less frequent IVC regimen for another 19 months and 10 years later, the patient is in good health and cancer-free.

Though we certainly can't call it a cure yet, IV vitamin C holds much promise and can certainly be used as an adjunct therapy in combination with other cancer treatments. And while you won't likely see it in mainstream oncologists' bag of tricks anytime soon, the good news is, there are clinics all over the world already using this incredible treatment and it's available right now. So if you or someone you love is suffering from cancer, IV vitamin C may be a worthy addition to your list of viable and promising treatment options.

CHAPTER 21

Finding the Cancer Cachexia Key

What if I told you that there is a drug out there right now that stops the progression of cancer in many patients, and the government has been keeping it from the American public for decades? The real-life story of this drug—hydrazine sulfate—is so dramatic, it will make you shudder at both the corruption of the medical establishment and the drastic implications for cancer treatment in the United States and around the world.

Hydrazine sulfate has been shown in human studies to improve and save lives *more than 50 percent of the time* and is used all over Russia in top cancer treatment programs. Incredibly, it's also cheaper than a pack of gum. In fact, it costs just three quarters of a cent per dose per day. So why haven't we heard more about this wonder drug? Well, I'm sure there's no need for me to reiterate the most common motive for the suppression of inexpensive cancer treatments—let's just say that two-thirds of oncologists' income comes from the sale of chemotherapy drugs to patients. But, I digress!

Back to the amazing story of hydrazine sulfate...

Fueling the Search for a Cancer Cure

Dr. Joseph Gold began his career with a great passion to find the biochemical cause of cancer. After his post-doctorate studies at UC Berkley, Dr. Gold was inducted into the U.S. Air Force and spent three years in the Mercury Astronaut selection program. After leaving the program with a citation from President Eisenhower for his work, Dr. Gold turned his attention to a new goal: Finding the medicine that could stop the weight loss and debilitation from which cancer patients suffer. Despite what we've been led to believe, this wasting away—a condition called cachexia—is what actually kills most cancer patients. In fact, it accounts for 73 percent of all cancer deaths.

While it was commonly thought that the syndrome only occurs late in the disease, Dr. Gold discovered that cachexia begins bio-

Understanding Cachexia

In a chronic disease like cancer, cachexia causes the appetite to diminish, until the patient ultimately develops anorexia. Since the body still needs nourishment, it begins to break down its fat and protein stores, via a process called gluconeogenesis, for the body to use as energy. The glucose metabolism of a tumor and/or cancer cell is much less efficient than that of a normal cell; normal cells metabolize glucose (sugar) aerobically, using oxygen, which is 15 times more efficient than cancer cells, which metabolize glucose anaerobically through a process of fermentation. Fermentation, being less efficient, requires much more sugar and since the metabolic rate of a tumor is much higher than that of a normal cell anyway, the amount of sugar needed is even greater. This sugar is derived from body breakdown products. Eventually the patient dies trying to feed the tumor, which is why cachexia is the major cause of death in cancer patients.[2]

chemically with *the very first cancer cell.* And stopping it is absolutely critical in winning the war on cancer.

But, according to Dr. Gold "the trouble with cachexia [was] no one knew anything about how it came about. It was a complete mystery."[1]

So Dr. Gold continued his research and found that if a certain enzyme called PEPCK could be inhibited, cancer cachexia could theoretically be stopped. Not long after his theory was developed, Dr. Gold found himself at a conference on enzymes where another group of researchers were giving a presentation on a chemical that could inhibit the very same PEPCK enzyme. The chemical was called hydrazine sulfate, a natural compound used in a number of different industrial processes, including the production of rocket fuel.[1]

Research and NCI Suppression: A Matter of Ego and Economics

It didn't take long after these two big discoveries for hydrazine sulfate to become the subject of controlled clinical trials around the world. There were three main sets of studies done on the compound: those conducted at the Petrov Research Institute of Oncology in St Petersburg, Russia, those done at the Harbor-UCLA Medical Center in L.A., and those sponsored by the U.S. National Cancer Institute (NCI).

The 17 years of Russian studies—all published in U.S., peer-reviewed cancer journals— and the 10 years of UCLA studies (also published in prestigious medical journals) showed amazing efficacy and safety of hydrazine sulfate as a treatment for cancer cachexia. The only *inconsistent* results on hydrazine sulfate were from the studies conducted by the NCI.[1,3]

Unlike the Russian and UCLA studies, the studies done by the NCI all found hydrazine sulfate to be an ineffective treatment for cancer cachexia. So why did their results differ so greatly from the rest? The answer is that only the NCI-sponsored studies allowed subjects to take medications that were incompatible with the test drug.

Despite clear warnings against doing so, the NCI allowed the patients in their hydrazine sulfate studies to use of tranquilizers, barbituates, and alcohol. Hydrazine sulfate is actually a natural monoamine oxidase (MAO) inhibitor and compounds in this family are incompatible with drugs—like alcohol, tranquilizers, etc.—that suppress the central nervous system. In fact, if they're combined, these two substances can result in a potentially lethal interaction.

In essence, the NCI intentionally sabotaged the studies and succeeded in burying hydrazine sulfate for the next 20 years, issuing a paper stating that the drug was worthless. And, even worse, they put the lives of the study subjects at risk in the process!

Why would the NCI deliberately sabotage hydrazine sulfate as a treatment for cancer? As you've probably guessed already, the answer is most likely money-related. Pharmaceutical-grade hydrazine sulfate costs only three-quarters of one cent per dose—so it goes without saying that cancer doctors would not make a lot of money off this drug.

Benefits of Using Hydrazine Sulfate

But profitable for drug companies and oncologists or not, hydrazine sulfate helps cancer patients significantly. Controlled clinical trials indicate approximately half of all patients who take hydrazine sulfate experience weight gain, restored appetite, extended survival time, and a major reduction in pain and suffering, which are critical benefits for those in the midst of the cancer battle. Many patients also report feeling more vigorous and that

Raisins and 15 Other Foods to Avoid During Hydrazine Sulfate Therapy

MAO inhibitors are most commonly known for their anti-depressant effects, but they also have another important job in the body—breaking down the amino acid tyramine.

When you're taking an MAO inhibitor, eating foods that contain tyramine can cause blood pressure and heart rate to skyrocket, which leads to headaches, or much worse symptoms. To complicate things even further, hydrazine sulfate is actually inactivated by tyramine. As a result, for those thinking of taking hydrazine sulfate, a tyramine-free diet is an absolute must.

Foods that contain tyramine include

- all cheeses, except cottage cheese and cream cheese
- dried and cured meats (ex: bologna, salami, etc.)
- pickled herring and salted dried fish
- meat extracts
- yeast extracts/brewer's yeast
- all alcoholic beverages
- pickles, sauerkraut
- fruits: avocados, canned figs, raisins, bananas
- cultured dairy products
- fermented soy (miso)
- beef or chicken liver

In general, high-protein foods that have undergone aging should be avoided. Also, avoid any over-the-counter cold or allergy remedy.[2]

many symptoms disappear, along with more feelings of well-being.

But even more importantly, large-scale clinical trials suggest that hydrazine sulfate affects every type of tumor at every stage.

Studies at UCLA and at the Petrov Institute showed that the most frequent side effects (which occurred in less than 10 percent of the cases) were nausea and vomiting, but that as soon as the dosage was lowered, these side effects disappeared. There was no evidence of organ damage or damage to the immunological defense system as usually occurs with conventional chemotherapy.[3]

Hydrazine sulfate can be used safely with radiation, too. According to Dr. Gold, the use of hydrazine sulfate and radiation together results in a "synergistic effect" and because there are two different mechanisms of anti-cancer action operating, [the combination] is...tremendously effective for tumors that otherwise have no effective treatment."

The Future of Hydrazine Sulfate

The controlled clinical trials thus far show a 46 percent benefit in late-stage patients that haven't responded to anything else. Dr. Gold asserts that with hydrazine sulfate "many will have a stabilized condition or regression for two months or longer—and many have gone years, stabilized, and some will go on to long term cure."

Fortunately, hydrazine sulfate's long battle is drawing to a close—and it has emerged victorious. This tremendous breakthrough is no longer considered an "unconventional therapy" and is actually medically available right now—even in the U.S.. According to Dr. Gold "the best way [to access it] is to have a licensed physician write a prescription for it and the prescription filled at a compounding pharmacy."

Of course, if you are thinking about using hydrazine sulfate yourself, be sure to check with your doctor first.

CHAPTER 22

Citrus Peels Provide Powerful Cancer Protection

Next time somebody offers you a glass of zesty lemonade or a cup of tea with a twist, you may want to take them up on their offer—and ask for refills, too. It turns out that the peels of citrus fruits like lemons, oranges, and grapefruit, contain a compound called d-limonene. And studies are showing that it's got powerful protective activity against a variety of cancers. Although it's still early in the game and Phase II clinical trials are just beginning, limonene already appears to hold great promise for cancer treatment.

A Drop of Citrus History

Though we don't know their exact origin, most researchers believe citrus fruits came from Southeast Asia at least 4,000 years BC. Citrus fruits were first taken to North Africa and then to Southern Europe where they flourished in the Middle Ages, before being brought to America by the Spaniards and the Portuguese.

Citrus fruits belong to the Rutaceae family and their evergreen trees give fruits of different forms and sizes which are full of fragrance, flavor, and juice—and it's their juicy inside pulp that's rich in sugars, vitamin C, pectin, fibers, different organic acids and potassium salt, which is what gives them their characteristic flavor. In terms of nutrition, we all know that citrus fruits and juices are rich in vitamin C as well as folic acid, and they're a good source of fiber too. Citrus also contains potassium, calcium, thiamin, niacin, vitamin B6, phosphorus, magnesium, and copper.[1, 2]

Back to the Rind

While the inside flesh of citrus fruits contains a lot of nutritional value, it's the peels that have made recent headlines, thanks to their d-limonene content. D-limonene is known as a dietary monoterpene, a chemical group which scientists have known to possess anti-tumor activities for some time now. Limonene specifically has been shown in rats to be particularly active against breast, skin, liver, lung, pancreatic and stomach cancers.[1] But how does it actually work inside our cells to combat cancer?

Well, there are several theories, but studies are pointing in the direction of induction of cancer cell apoptosis or "cell suicide." It also seems to inhibit the ability of cancer cells to communicate with each other.[3]

While studies are still in the works to pinpoint the exact mechanism, some very positive research has emerged on limonene already, such as a 1996 study which found that limonene reduces the growth of pancreatic cancer cells by a whopping *50 percent.*[4] Another study on a breast cancer patient who was taking a dose of 8 grams twice daily for 11 months, plus three additional patients with colorectal cancer who were taking .5 or 1 gram of d-limonene twice daily, all showed disease stabilization for longer than six months after taking it.[5]

Yet another recent study from University of Arizona found that consuming citrus peel can reduce the risk of skin cancer by 30 percent. And when it is consumed with hot black tea, the risk of skin cancer is reduced by more than 70 percent. Additional lab tests concluded that d-limonene, reduces not only the incidence and size of tumors at several sites, but also the growth of various tumor cells.[6]

So how much limonene do you need to take? As it stands now, the recommendation is 7.3 to 14.4 grams per day.[5,6]

10 Tasty Ways to Get Your Limonene

Studies indicate that as little as 1 tablespoon of citrus zest per week is enough to make a significant difference in your cancer risk. One tablespoon of zest is equivalent to the peel of approximately one orange or lemon, depending on the size of the fruit and how finely or coarsely the zest is grated. Here are some suggestions for adding it to your diet:

- Prepare lemonade from the whole fruit, including the peel
- Use grated lemon or grapefruit zest as a salad topping along with a sprinkling of pecans or walnuts
- Mix some lemon zest into your salsa
- Sprinkle grated orange and lemon zest on top of chicken or fish
- Add lemon zest to your tea
- Grate citrus peels into cottage cheese
- Candy the citrus peels and use in baking
- Top hot tomato soup or gazpacho with grated lemon peel
- Add lemon zest to fruit compote
- Mix orange peel into your cranberry sauce on Thanksgiving (or any day of the year!)

When Life Gives You Lemons...

There's no doubt that limonene is quite worthy of its place in the ever-expanding list of promising cancer treatments, and I, for one, am excited to see what the continued research on it will bring to light. And while we wait, I see no reason why we shouldn't all take advantage of this gift from Mother Nature, who surely knows best, and incorporate limonene into our every day lives as both a cancer preventative and a sweet spice of life.

Limonene softgel supplements are available though www.lef.org and www.iherb.com.

CHAPTER 23

Packing a Powerful Anti-Cancer Punch with Paw Paw

A cousin of graviola (see chapter 3), the American Paw Paw has been the subject of research for 25 years now because of its variety of cancer-curing compounds called acetogenins. Dr. Jerry McLaughlin of Purdue University has published over 100 articles and studies on the health benefits of acetogenins, which have been found to regulate the production of energy in cancer cells and reduce the growth of the blood vessels that nourish cancerous tumors.

In addition, Paw Paw is also one of the only cancer treatments that has shown any effectiveness against multiple drug-resistant (MDR) cells, which is key in keeping cancer from coming back. Research has also shown that Paw Paw compounds are up to 300 times more potent than Taxol (a chemo drug used to treat breast cancer) and can even help prevent cachexia. With all of this great stuff going for it, I just had to dig up some more on Paw Paw for you, and here's what else I found out...

And the Research Says...

Paw Paw is unique mostly because of its special carbon chains called Annonaceous acetogenins. While all plants with acetogenins have certain features in common, Paw Paw's molecules in particular have been studied by extensively by Dr. McLaughlin and his team at Purdue University, as well as many other researchers, who have spent years uncovering their chemical structures and testing them for their anti-cancer properties. But unlike a lot of cancer research that's often kept a trade secret, Dr McLaughlin's research has been freely disseminated since the moment he began.[(2)]

As I've already mentioned, there's a lot of great research out there already on the amazing Paw Paw. In a 1997 issue of Cancer Letters, it was explained that an acetogenin in Paw Paw called bullatacin is seriously toxic to multidrug-resistant (MDR) human breast cancer cells and has a special advantage in the chemotherapeutic treatment of certain MDR tumors.[(3)] Another 1997 study on the relationship between Annonaceous acetogenins and MDR breast cancer cells found that 14 diverse acetogenins in Paw Paw inhibited the growth of breast cancer cells resistant to treatment with three types of chemo drugs. In fact, the acetogenins in Paw Paw had 250 times the potency of one of the most common forms of chemo, adriamycin.[(4)]

Most recently, in 2008 the Journal of Natural Products published an article on Paw Paw stating that its extracts are among the most potent of the 3,500 species of plants screened for bioactive compounds at Purdue University.[(5)]

The four main ways that Paw Paw battles cancer are:

1. It slows and blocks the production of cell energy in abnormal cells

2. It prevents the growth of blood vessels in or near tumors

3. It depletes the DNA building blocks necessary for new, abnormal cell division

4. It can kill cells that are resistant to chemotherapy and keep cancer away for good[1]

Destroying Indestructible Cells

Approximately 2 percent of most tumors are made up of multiple drug-resistant cells against which chemo is not effective. These MDR cells resist chemo by turning on a pump that takes the medicine right out of the cancer cells. In theory, if the first round of chemo is a success, then all of the cells that are not MDR are destroyed. And since they make up the vast majority of the tumor mass, in theory, the tumor will appear to have been effectively destroyed.

But, often, the MDR cells start to multiply and form a new tumor that is made up entirely of MDR cells, so when chemo is used again, none of the cells will be able to be destroyed like the first time.

And Paw Paw is the only cancer treatment that has shown effectiveness against MDR cells.[6]

Paw Paw gravitates toward cells that use a lot of energy and cuts off their energy supply. Since cancer cells use 10-17 times the energy of a normal cell, Paw Paw acts on these cancer cells with great efficacy. But if there's no cancer, parasite, or other major energy consuming cells in your body, Paw Paw can head for the fast-growing cells lining your intestinal walls, and cause a stomachache, which is why long-term use is not advised (and certainly pregnant women should never use it). To prevent digestive distress such as nausea, always take Paw Paw with food and always check in with your doctor before adding it to your protocol.[6]

There are some other substances that increase ATP energy (a cell's energy currency) and should therefore be avoided when taking Paw Paw:

- Hydrogen peroxide
- Vitamin C
- Vitamin E
- Co-Q10
- Thyroid support products
- L-cysteine
- N-acetylsteine
- Glutathione
- Burdock Root
- Essiac and Flor-Essence (see chapter 19)
- Ozone treatments (hyperbaric oxygen is acceptable)
- Flax seed oil
- Grapefruit seed extract (due to high vitamin C content)
- Whey protein

If you want to try Paw Paw, look for the standardized Paw Paw Twig Extract (Asimina triloba) by Healthy Sunshine. You can contact them by calling (888)523-1727 or visit www.healthy-sunshine.com.

CHAPTER 24

The Citrus Secret Stopping Metastasis in Its Tracks

It looks like the citrus family has another surprise in store for us...The latest research shows that a substance called modified citrus pectin (MCP), commonly used as a gelling agent for canning foods and making jellies, may be the next cancer-fighting all-star.

In the past 10 years, research on MCP's effectiveness in blocking metastasis (spreading) of certain types of cancers, including melanomas, prostate, and breast cancers has skyrocketed. And it looks like this incredible citrus peel compound may have the potential to stop your cancer from spreading—and maybe even wipe it out for good.

Peeling Away Cancer Cells' Power

Pectin is a carbohydrate that's made of thousands of sugar molecules that are chemically linked together. It's found in most plants and is particularly plentiful in the peels of apples, citrus fruits, and plums. Modified citrus pectin (MCP) is a form of pectin that's been chemically altered to be more easily absorbed by the digestive tract by breaking its molecules into smaller pieces. Pectin that has not been modified cannot be absorbed from the digestive system (and is considered a type of soluble dietary fiber), whereas modified pectin can be absorbed right into the bloodstream.[1]

So where does MCP come into the cancer story? Well, in order for cancer cells to spread, or metastasize, they must first clump together, and it's the galectins on their surface which are thought to be responsible for much of this clumping potential. Research shows that modified citrus pectin is particularly rich in a sugar called galactose, which likes to bind to the surface of cancer cells, and as a result MCP can block cancer cells from grouping together and spreading.[2]

Because metastasis is so life-threatening, most research on anti-metastatic therapies has either been done using in vitro (test tube) cell cultures or animal studies, and although it's still unclear exactly how these study results translate to humans, the results are quite promising thus far.[3]

Research Maps Out MCP's Potential

Though it's just the beginning, we've already got quite a bit of research available on MCP and I've gathered some of the best of it right here for you:

A 2007 study published in the journal Oncology examined the clinical benefits of MCP in patients with advanced solid tumors. The researchers found that 20.7 percent of the patients taking MCP had an overall clinical benefit, 22.5 percent showed a stabilized disease, and 12.5 percent were stable for longer than 24 weeks with the MCP treatment.[4]

Another study examined MCP's effectiveness against prostate cancer metastasis in rats and found that while the oral MCP did not affect primary tumor growth, it significantly reduced metastases when compared to control animals.[5]

A human study examined the effect of MCP on prostate specific antigen (PSA) doubling time in seven prostate cancer patients (PSA is an enzymatic tumor marker and its doubling time tends to reflect the speed at which the cancer is growing). They found that four of seven patients exhibited more than 30-percent lengthening of PSA doubling time.[6]

Research has shown that breast cancer metastasis requires clumping and binding of the cancerous cells to outer tissue layers in order for it to actually invade the neighboring tissue.[7] But when MCP was studied in vitro against breast carcinoma cell lines, the researchers found that MCP blocked the adhesion of malignant cells to blood vessel endothelia (the sensitive, innermost lining of blood vessels), thus inhibiting metastasis.[8]

A final study done in mice determined that MCP significantly decreased tumor metastasis to the lung by more than 90 percent.[9]

MCP Dosing

These results are pretty exciting and I know you're probably wondering how to find MCP and how to take it. Well, citrus pectin is actually on the FDA's list of ingredients that are "generally recognized as safe" or GRAS. I know that I, for one, am pretty excited to see that there's a potential alternative cancer treatment out there that the FDA is not clamping down on like they usually do.

Modified citrus pectin is available in capsules or a powder and the typically recommended dose for the powder is 5 grams (about $1/_5$ of an ounce) mixed with water or juice and taken three times a day with meals. For capsules, the suggested dose is 800 milligrams (mg) 3 times a day with meals.[10] When it's used as intended there are rarely side effects (some people may experience stomach discomfort after taking MCP, and there have been a few cases of people with exposure to powdered pectin developing asthma when the pectin was inhaled during use, so don't take MCP if you're allergic to citrus).

MCP is available as PectaSol C Modified Citrus Pectin by Econugenics, Inc. You can contact Econugenics by calling (800) 308-5518 or visit www.econugenics.com.

CHAPTER 25

The Cutting Edge of Cancer Treatment: Immunotherapies from Around the World

I've spent quite a bit of time now delving into the wide array of cancer cures being used across the globe and what I've found is that the old saying is true: "there's more than one way to skin a cat."

There are plenty of effective alternative cancer treatments out there to choose from, being used right now on each and every continent, and there's one thing that many of them have in common: they help repair the cancer elimination job that our immune systems haven't done right in the first place. My recent talk with Dr. Sean Devlin has shown me just that—that immune-boosting indeed may be the future of cancer treatment in both the conventional and alternative worlds.

Dr. Sean Devlin, who is based in Colorado and works in a number of clinics throughout the U.S., has been working with two cutting-edge cancer doctors, Dr. Tsuneo Kobayoshi from Japan and Dr. Meredith Rigdon Lentz from Germany. Both doctors use immunotherapy, or the stimulation of the immune system to reject and destroy tumors, in the treatment of cancer—and their patient waiting lists are growing wildly. News of these treatments is only recently getting out in the U.S., and I'm pretty sure this is one of the first places you're going to hear of them...

New Advances Track Your Progress Every Step of the Way

One of the biggest roadblocks in cancer treatment is assessing exactly how much progress a patient has made in terms of healing, and if in remission, what the biological signs are that the cancer may be coming back. Dr. Tsuneo Kobayoshi has invented a way to analyze a variety of tumor markers in an effort to gauge how well a person is doing pre-, during, and post-cancer care, whether being treated with traditional, integrative, or a combination of therapies.

Dr. Devlin explained that Dr. Kobayoshi's testing program involves about 17 different tumor markers that he uses to measure and classify his patients into five categories: 1 being low risk for dying from a cancer-associated illness, and 5 being a highly severe prognosis. Many people get these markers done in order to determine whether to go into a preventative program or to check whether their conventional cancer treatment has really left them free of cancer.

But regardless of your classification, you can use Dr. Kobayoshi's techniques to stimulate your immune system to fight or prevent cancer. The first thing Dr. Kobayoshi recommends is to make it difficult for cancer cells to thrive in the body by following an alkalinizing, low-sugar diet (cancer cells thrive on sugar), and taking a few specific herbal supplements and intravenous sodium bicarbonate (see chapter 6).

He also stimulates the immune system to fight the cancer off with a diluted version of Coley's vaccine, which is a mixture of

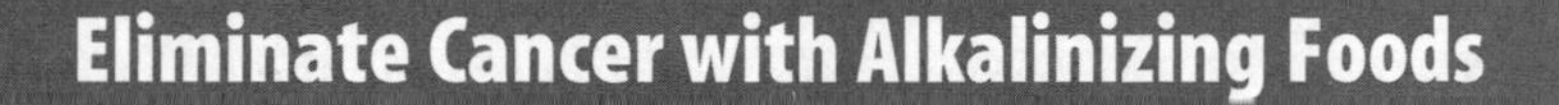

Eliminate Cancer with Alkalinizing Foods

Here is a brief list of alkaline foods you can eat to help keep cancer away:

- Dark green and yellow vegetables and root vegetables
- Fresh vegetable juices
- Soaked nuts like almonds or hazelnuts
- Sprouted grains and beans like alfalfa, mung beans, clover and radish
- Essential fatty acids from flax oil, borage oil, and virgin olive oil
- Soy products like tofu
- Seaweed
- Onions and garlic
- Add lemon zest to fruit compote
- Fruits like avocados, lemons, limes and grapefruits(2)

dead bacteria. Their presence in the body helps kick the immune system into high gear by causing a high fever.

Taking Matters into Your Own Hands

While Dr. Kobayoshi's therapies stimulate the body's immune system to help itself, Dr. Meredith Rigdon Lentz's approach is to get in and do the immune system's work for it.

About 20 years ago, Dr. Lentz conducted a series of studies on pregnant goats in attempt to find the origin of cancer and how it develops. The research uncovered an important protective mechanism within the goats' fetuses which allowed them to protect themselves from their mother's immune system (otherwise the mother's body will reject the growing baby, considering it a "foreign invader). This protective mechanism defends the fetus against immune cell products called cytokines in the mother's system (which include tumor necrosis factor or TNF, interleukins, and interferons).

Dr. Lentz hypothesized that, like the goat fetuses, the cancer cells in our bodies had found a way to resist our cytokines by sending out receptors into the blood to stop them. Amazingly, Dr. Lentz was able to create a device, somewhat similar to a kidney dialysis machine, which filters out all of these receptors, allowing our cytokines to do their job and stop cancer in its tracks. Dr. Lentz originally worked on getting approval for the device in the U.S., but the FDA made it virtually impossible. Today, Dr. Lentz treats patients from all over the world, but only in Germany.

Help Here at Home

I know what you're thinking: These treatments sound incredible, but where do I go for the cutting edge cancer treatment if I'm not in Germany or Japan? Well, I would suggest heading straight to Dr. Devlin, who uses an integrative approach, combining alternative and conventional treatments to treat cancer.

Dr. Devlin also encourages the use of biofeedback, acupuncture, and homeopathy. And Dr. Devlin is also working hard to bring Dr. Kobayoshi's and Dr. Lentz's therapies to patients here in the U.S.

You can contact Dr. Devlin by calling (530)274-2274 or visiting www.highlandspringswellness.com

CHAPTER 26

Giving Patients a Shot at a Cancer-Free Future

What if the cure for cancer was as simple as year's worth of weekly shots at the doctor's office? Sounds far-fetched, but such an incredible option may be just around the bend.

Dr. Nobuto Yamamoto, director of the Division of Cancer Immunology and Molecular Biology at the Socrates Institute for Therapeutic Immunology in Philadelphia, has discovered a way to increase the levels of a certain glycoprotein (a compound which contains a sugar and protein component) in your bloodstream, whose role is to activate macrophages to kill tumor cells.

You see, normally when this glycoprotein, called Gc protein (also called vitamin D binding protein) is converted to its active form, Gc-MAF, it activates the macrophage cells of the immune system to kill off foreign invaders like viruses and bacteria—and, in theory, cancer too.

However, since tumor cells secrete an enzyme called nagalase that blocks the conversion of Gc to Gc-NAF, macrophages are actually prevented from carrying out their role as a cancer hit-man.

Incredibly, Dr. Yamamoto may have found a way around the nagalase enzyme problem. In his recent study published in the International Journal of Cancer, Dr. Yamamoto found that after 16 subjects with breast cancer received weekly doses of Gc-NAF for 16 to 22 weeks, the nagalase enzyme secreted by tumors fell to normal levels, indicating that *their tumors had been eliminated.*[1]

In a follow up study on eight patients with colon cancer, all experienced the disappearance of tumors after 32 to 50 injections, with no recurrence in the next seven years.

A year's worth of shots might sound like a pain (literally and figuratively), but when you consider the months of agonizing chemotherapy and radiation that so many cancer patients have to endure, the idea suddenly becomes a lot more enticing...

So could this be one of the latest and greatest in our cancer bag of cures? Well, the initial results are very exciting, but larger and more comprehensive studies are definitely in order. But we've also got to remember that Gc-NAF is a naturally occurring molecule, and, as we well know, what cannot be patented doesn't draw in Big Pharma's big bucks to fund the necessary studies...So until that changes, we may have to sit back and wait for Gc-NAF's big emergence to the world of cancer cures.

References

Know the Enemy

[1] http://www.who.int/mediacentre/factsheets/fs297/en/index.html

[2] http://abcnews.go.com/Nightline/Story?id=3623642&page=1

[3] http://www.organicconsumers.org/foodsafety/cancercure050405.cfm

[4] http://www.cancer.gov/cancertopics/factsheet/detection/staging

[5] Proctor, Robert. Cancer Wars: How Politics Shapes What We Know and Don't Know About Cancer. New York: Basic Books, 1995, p. 4. See: http://curezone.com/diseases/cancer/cancer_radiation_therapy.asp

[6] Gottlieb S, "Chemotherapy may be overused at the end of life," BMJ 2001; 322: 1,267. See: http://www.rense.com/general81/chemo.htm

[7] Fisher B, et al. "Postoperative Radiotherapy in the Treatment of Breast Cancer; Results of the NSAPP Clinical Trial," Annals of Surgery 1970; 172(4)

[8] http://www.fwhc.org/health/nocure.htm

[9] www.cancer.org

[10] http://www.aflcio.org/aboutus/thisistheaflcio/publications/ magazine/0503_bigfix.cfm

[11] http://www.cancertutor.com/WarBetween/War_Fda.html

[12] http://curezone.com/art/read.asp?ID=91&db=5&C0=779

BEC-5: The Eggplant Cure from Down Under

[1] http://www.vanuatumedical.com/cham_interview

[2] Cham BE, Daunter B, Evans RA. "Topical treatment of malignant and premalignant skin lesions by very low concentrations of a standard mixture (BEC) of solasodine alkaloids." Cancer Letters 1991; 59: 183-192

[3] Cerio R, Punjabi S. (Dermatology Department, 2nd floor Outpatient Building, Royal London Hospital, Whitechapel, London E1 188. Telephone 020 7377 7000.) "Clinical Appraisal of BEC5." Letter dated April 23, 2002

Graviola: A Fruitful Gift from the Amazon

[1] http://www.hsibaltimore.com/articles/hsi_2001ds/ hsi_200101_awb9.html

[2] http://www.rain-tree.com/graviola.htm

[3] J Nat Prod 1995; 58(6):902-908

[4] Rieser MJ, Gu ZM, Fang XP, et al. "Five novel mono-tetrahydrofuran ring acetogenins from the seeds of Annona muricata." J Nat Prod 1996; 59(2): 100-8

[5] Anticancer Res 1998; 18(1A): 119-24

(6) Proc Natl Acad Sci USA 1996; 93(16): 8,618-23

(7) Anticancer Res 1992; 12(3): 837-43

Ancient Anti-Cancer Herbal from the Orient: Chinese Happy Tree

(1) http://www.herbs2000.com/herbs/herbs_xi_shu.htm

(2) Journal of the American Chemical Society 1966: 88; 3,888. See: http://pubs.acs.org/cen/acsnews/8120/8120acsnews.html

(3) http://www.hmcboston.com/HCC/Herbal%20Therapy/DOC/ Injectable%20Herbs.doc

(4) http://davesgarden.com/guides/articles/view/206/

SIDEBAR: The Natural Pharmacist (www.tnp.com), "Healthy Healing," 11th edition by Linda Page, Alternatives from Nature (www.herbsrainbear.com), www.Herbwalk.com www.Healthphone.com, www.Holisticonline.com.

Dr. Budwig's Biochemical Balancer: Flax oil and Cottage Cheese Diet

(1) http://www.cancertutor.com/Cancer/Budwig.html

(2) http://www.umm.edu/altmed/articles/flaxseed-oil-000304.htm

(3) http://www.cancer.org/docroot/ETO/content/ ETO_5_3x_Flaxseed.asp

(4) http://curezone.com/foods/flaxseed_oil.html

(5) http://www.cancure.org/budwig_diet.htm

(6) http://www.healingcancernaturally.com/budwigtestimonials.rtf

Dynamic Alkalinizing Duo: Cesium Chloride & DMSO

(1) http://www.cancer-coverup.com/brewer/printbrewerreport.htm

(2) http://alternativecancer.us/cesiumchloride.htm

(3) http://www.alternative-cancer-care.com/Cesium_Chloride.html

(4) http://www.newswithviews.com/Howenstine/james14.htm

(5) http://www.doaj.org/doaj?func=abstract&id=183432&toc=y

A Nutrition Revolution: Dr. Gerson's Cancer Detox Diet

(1) www.gerson.org

(2) Fischer, William. How to Fight Cancer and Win. Baltimore: Agora Health Books, 1992.

(3) http://cancer-research.net/GersonPubs.html

(4) http://www.gerson.org/g_therapy/mg.asp

(5) http://www.cancer.gov/cancertopics/pdq/cam/gerson/Patient/ ▯
page2/print

(6) Robbins J. Reclaiming Our Health: Exploding the Medical Myth and Embracing the Source. Tiburon, CA: HJ Kramer, 1998
See: http://books.google.com/books?id=4NftA-D9xr8C&pg= ▯
PA280&lpg=PA280&dq=max+gerson+and+AMA&source= ▯
web&ots=vKki9tqPEo&sig=CP-k3xVnxR1Vppp4AZb1z2CeVo0&hl= ▯
en&sa=X&oi=book_result&resnum=10&ct=result#PPA280,M1)

(7) Hildenbrand, et al. "Five year survival rates of melanoma patients treated by diet therapy after the manner of Gerson." Altern Ther Health Med 1995:1(4); 29-37

(8) http://www.gersonplus.com/soup.html

(9) Molassiotis A, Peat P. "Surviving against all odds: Analysis of 6 case studies of patients with cancer who followed Gerson Therapy." Integr Cancer Ther 2007: 6(1); 80-8

(10) http://rawfoodstips.com/

(11) http://www.living-foods.com/recipes/lettucewraps.html

More than Just a Christmas Kiss: Wiping Out Cancer with Mistletoe

(1) "Mistletoe as a treatment for cancer," BMJ 2006; 333: 1,282-3

(2) http://www.cancer.gov/cancertopics/pdq/cam/mistletoe/ patient/Page2

(3) http://www.hsibaltimore.com/ealerts/ea200106/ea20010607.html

(4) "Mistletoe in cancer - a systematic review on controlled clinical trials." Eur J Med Res 2003; 8(3):109-19

(5) "Iscador/Mistletoe in the treatment of cancer," Cancer Cure Foundation (cancure.org)

(6) http://usa.weleda.com/medicine/ medical_practitioner_center/index.aspx

Kick Out Carcinogens with Curcumin

(1) http://www.lionsgrip.com/curhistory.htm

(2) Anticancer Res 2002; 22(6C): 4,179-81

(3) http://www.chinaphar.com/1671-4083/28/423.htm

(4) Inano H, Onoda M, Inafuku N, et al. "Potent preventative action

of curcumin on radiation-induced initiation of mammary tumorigenesis in rats." Carcinogenesis 2000; 18: 83-8.

(5) Aggarwal BB. "Curcumin Suppresses the Paclitaxel-Induced Nuclear Factor-ÃªB Pathway in Breast Cancer Cells and Inhibits Lung Metastasis of Human Breast Cancer in Nude Mice." Clin Canc Res; 11(20): 7,490-98

(6) Seo KI, Choi MS, Jung UJ, et al. "Effect of curcumin supplementation on blood glucose, plasma insulin, and glucose homeostasis related enzyme activities in diabetic db/db mice." Mol Nutr Food Res 2008; 52(9): 995-1,004

Triphala: Ayurveda's Triumphant Cancer-Fighting Trio

(1) Sandhya T, et al. "Potential of traditional ayurvedic formulation, Triphala, as a novel anticancer drug." Cancer Letters 2006; 231(2): 206-14

(2) http://www.indolink.com/displayArticleS.php?id=082106115647

(3) http://www.scienceblog.com/cms/
triphala-hinders-growth-pancreatic-cancer-cells-13041.html

(4) http://www.planetherbs.com/articles/triphala.html

Killing the Fungus Among Us: Dr. Simoncini's Sodium Bicarbonate Treatment

(1) http://www.curenaturalicancro.com/2-why-people-die-cancer.html

(2) Interview with Doug Kaufmann http://www.know-the-cause.com/
Shows/TullioSimonciniMDWithDougKaufmann/tabid/
109/Default.aspx

(3) Karthaus M. "Treatment of fungal infections led to leukemia remissions." Sept. 28, 1999

(4) Medical Hypotheses 1996; 47: 35-38

(5) http://www.oardc.ohio-state.edu/ohiofieldcropdisease/ Mycotoxins/mycopagedefault.htm

(6) http://www.townsendletter.com/Dec2007/ltr_cancerfungus1207.htm

(7) http://www.cancertutor.com/faq/faq_inexpensive.html

(8) http://www.healingcancernaturally.com/ sodium-bicarbonate-treatment.html

Staying Balanced and Cancer-Free With Macrobiotics

(1) http://www.cancer.org/docroot/ETO/content/ ETO_5_3X_Macrobiotic_Diet.asp

(2) http://xnet.kp.org/permanentejournal/fall02/macrobiotic.html

(3) http://www.pccnaturalmarkets.com/health/1297003/

(4) Carter JP, et al. "Hypothesis: Dietary Management May Improve Survival from Nutritionally Linked Cancers Based on Analysis of Representative Cases," Journal of the American College of Nutrition 1993: 12: 209-226

(5) Kagawa Y. "Impact of Westernization on the Nutrition of Japan," Preventive Medicine 1978; 7: 205-17.

(6) http://altmedicine.about.com/od/popularhealthdiets/a/ Macrobiotic.htm

(7) http://articles.mercola.com/sites/articles/archive/2001/07/28/ macrobiotics.aspxhttp://www.shareguide.com/Kushi.html

(8) http://www.cancerproject.org/ask/macrobiotic.php

Laetrile: Nature's Secret Cancer-Fighting Vitamin

(1) Krebs ET Jr. "The Nitrilosides in plants and animals," from Vitamin B17. New Rochelle: Arlington House, 1974, p.145-64. See: http://www.smart-drugs.com/ias-laetrile-cancer.htm

(2) http://www.laetrile.com.au/copy.asp?sect=q1&page=howdoes

(3) http://cancertutor.com/Cancer/Laetrile.html

(4) http://www.smart-drugs.com/ias-laetrile-cancer.htm

(5) Culbert, M. What the Medical Establishment Won't Tell You That Could Save Your Life. Virginia Beach: Donning Co., 1983. See: http://www.smart-drugs.com/ias-laetrile-cancer.htm

(6) http://alternativecancer.us/laetrile.htm

(7) http://www.cancure.org/laetrile.htm

(8) http://findarticles.com/p/articles/mi_m0ISW/ ▯
is_2002_June/ai_86387541

(9) "Study says Laetrile not effective as Cancer Cure," The New York Times, May 1, 1981.
See: http://query.nytimes.com/gst/fullpage.html?sec= ▯
health&res=9E04E1D91638F932A35756C0A967948260

(10) The Ultimate Guide to B17 Metabolic Therapy Book. See: www.worldwithoutcancer.org.uk

An Endangered Medicine from the Taiwanese Mountains: Antrodia camphorata

(1) Hsiao G, Shen MY, Lin KH, et al. "Antioxidative and hepatoprotective effects of Antrodia camphorata extract." J Agric Food Chem 2003; 51(11): 3,302-8

[2] Hsu YL, Kuo YC, Kuo PL, et al. "Apoptotic effects of extract from Antrodia camphorata fruiting bodies in human hepatocellular carcinoma cell lines." Cancer Lett. 2005; 221(1): 77-89

[3] Song TY, Hsu SL, Yen GC. "Induction of apoptosis in human hepatoma cells by mycelia of Antrodia camphorate in submerged culture." J Ethnopharmacol 2005; 100(1-2): 158-67

[4] Peng CC, Chen KC, Peng RY, et al. "Antrodia camphorata extract induces replicative senescence in superficial TCC, and inhibits the absolute migration capability in invasive bladder carcinoma cells." J Ethnopharmacol 2007; 109(1): 93-103.

[5] Yang HL, Chen CS, Chang WH, et al. "Growth inhibition and induction of apoptosis in MCF-7 breast cancer cells by Antrodia camphorata." Cancer Lett. 2006; 231(2): 215-27.

[6] Liu JJ, Huang TS, Hsu ML, et al. "Antitumor effects of the partially purified polysaccharides from Antrodia camphorata and the mechanism of its action." Toxicol Appl Pharmacol 2004; 201(2): 186-93

[7] Wu H, Pan CL, Yao YC, et al. "Proteomic analysis of the effect of Antrodia camphorata extract on human lung cancer A549 cell." Proteomics 2006; 6(3): 826-35

[8] Chen CC, Shiao YJ, Lin RD, et al. "Neuroprotective diterpenes from the fruiting body of Antrodia camphorata." J Nat Prod 2006; 69(4): 689-91

Remedy from the Turkish Hillside: Nerium Oleander

[1] http://www.tbyil.com/oleander1.htm

[2] Anticancer Drugs 2000; 11(6): 455-63.

[3] http://www.naturalnews.com/023163.html

(4) http://www.cancertutor.com/Cancer02/Oleander.html

Albarin: The Incredible, Injectable Aloe Vera

(1) http://www.cancer.org/docroot/ETO/content/ETO_5_3x_Aloe.asp

(2) http://www.mskcc.org/mskcc/html/69116.cfm

(3) http://www.prlog.org/10000515-cancer-new-alternative-therapy.html

(4) http://www.naturalnews.com/021858.html

(5) Hammel, John C. "FDA Attacks Alternative Clinics-Cancer Patients' Lives Threatened," LEF, April 2002.

(6) http://www.altcancer.com/acemannan.htm

(7) http://www.serovera.com/contact.html

A New Frontier of Gene-Targeted Treatment: Dr. Burzynski and Antineoplaston Therapy

(1) Fischer, William. How to Fight Cancer and Win. Baltimore: Agora Health Books, 1992.

(2) Dr. Burzynski Interview Tape, April 2008

(3) www.burzynskiclinic.com

(4) http://www.commonweal.org/pubs/choices/21.html

(5) www.cancerhelp.org.uk

The Herbal Salve that Saved an Astronaut: The Story of Cansema

(1) Interview with Brian O'Leary, July 1, 2008

(2) Unpublished manuscript by Greg Caton

[3] http://health.centreforce.com/health/herbalhistory.html

[4] http://dev.m-w.com/dictionary/escharotics

[5] http://www.altcancer.com/can1.htm

[6] Interview with Greg Caton, April 2008

Essiac Tea: Nurse Caisse's Anti-Cancer Herbal Brew

[1] http://www.essiacinfo.org/

[2] http://www.healthfreedom.info/Cancer%20Essiac.htm

[3] Dombradi CA, Foldeak S. "Screening report on the antitumor activity of purified Arctium lappa extracts." Tumori 1966; 52: 173-6.

[4] Ottenweller J, et al. "Inhibition of prostate cancer-cell proliferation by Essiac." J Altern Complement Med 2004; 10(4): 687-91

[5] Kupchan SM, Karim A. "Tumor inhibitors: 114. Aloe emodin: antileukemic principle isolated from Rhamnus frangula L." Lloydia 1977; 39(4): 223-4

[6] Masuda T, Ueno Y. "Microsomal transformation of emodin into a direct mutagen." Mutat Res 1984; 125: 135-44.

[7] Russfield AB. "Pathology report. Project no C-114 [Essiac experiments]."Cambridge (MA): Biotech Research Consultants, 1959

[8] Wong CK, et al. "Immunomodulatory and anti-tumor polysaccharides from medicinal plants." J Int Med Res 1994; 22: 299-312

[9] Kennedy DA, et al. "In vitro analysis of herbal compound Essiac." Toronto, 2006.

[10] Blair, JN, et al. "An in vivo analysis of the herbal compound Essiac." Toronto, 2006.

[11] http://www.florahealth.com/Flora/Home/canada/Products/R8070.asp

Intravenous Vitamin C: Cancer-Killing Supervitamin

[1] http://www.nlm.nih.gov/medlineplus/ency/article/002404.htm

[2] Cameron E, Pauling L. "Supplemental Ascorbate in the supportive treatment of cancer: Prolongation of survival times in terminal human cancer." Proc Natl Acad Sci 1976; 73: 3,685-9

[3] Cameron E, Pauling L. "Supplemental Ascorbate in the supportive treatment of cancer: Re-evaluation of survival times in terminal human cancer." Proc Natl Acad Sci 1976; 75: 4,538-42

[4] Padayatty SJ, Levine M. "Reevaluation of Ascorbate in cancer treatment: Emerging evidence, Open minds and serendipity." J of Am Coll Nutr 2000; 19: 423-425

[5] http://www.townsendletter.com/Oct2004/warcancer1004.htm

[6] http://www.cmaj.ca/cgi/content/full/174/7/937

[7] http://www.orthomolecular.org/library/ivccancerpt.shtml

[8] "Intravenously Administered Vitamin C as Cancer Therapy: Three Cases" Canadian Medical Association Journal 2006; 174(7)

[9] www.nih.gov

Finding the Cancer Cachexia Key: Dr. Gold and Hydrazine Sulfate

[1] Interview with Dr. Gold, July 3, 2008

[2] http://cancertutor.com/Cancer/Hydrazine.html

[3] http://www.hydrazinesulfate.org/

[4] http://www.health-science-spirit.com/hydrazine.html

Citrus Peels Provide Powerful Cancer Protection with D-Limonene

[1] Crowell PL. "Prevention and Therapy of Cancer by Monoterpenes." J Nutr 1999: 129; 775S-778S.

[2] http://www.unctad.org/infocomm/anglais/orange/characteristics.htm

[3] http://www.mskcc.org/mskcc/html/69206.cfm

[4] http://www.lef.org/protocols/cancer/pancreatic_02.htm

[5] Vigushin DN, et al. "Phase I and pharmacokinetic study of D-Limonene in patients with advanced cancer. Cancer Research Campaign Phase I/II Clinical Trials Committee." Cancer Chemother Pharmacol 1998: 42; 111-7

[6] Hakim IA, Harris R, Ritenbaugh C. "Citrus Peel Use Is Associated With Reduced Risk of Squamous Cell Carcinoma of the Skin." Nutrition & Cancer 2000; 37(2): 43-50

[7] http://www.emedicine.com/emerg/topic511.htm

[8] http://www.mskcc.org/mskcc/html/69206.cfm

Packing a Powerful Anti-Cancer Punch with Paw Paw

[1] http://www.greatestherbsonearth.com/nsparticles/ pawpaw_cancer_remedy.htm

[2] http://www.mnwelldir.org/docs/cancer1/pawpaw.htm

[3] Cancer Letters 1997; 115: 73-9

[4] J Med Chem 1997; 40: 2,102-6

(5) http://www.ncbi.nlm.nih.gov/pubmed/18598079

(6) http://alternativecancer.us/pawpaw.htm

Stopping Metastasis in Its Tracks with Modified Citrus Pectin

(1) http://www.cancer.org/docroot/ETO/content/
ETO_5_3X_Modified_Citrus_Pectin.asp

(2) Strum S, Scholz M, McDermed J, et al. "Modified citrus pectin slows PSA doubling time: A pilot clinical trial." Presentation: International Conference on Diet and Prevention of Cancer, Tampere, Finland. May 28, 1999 - June 2, 1999. And Raz A, Loton R. "Endogenous galactoside-binding lectins: a new class of functional cell surface molecules related to metastasis." Cancer Metastasis Rev 1987; 6: 433-452

(3) http://findarticles.com/p/articles/mi_m0FDN/is_6_5/ai_68727255

(4) Azemar M, et al. "Clinical Benefit in Patients with Advanced Solid tumors treated with modified citrus pectin: A prospective pilot study." Oncology 2007: 1; 73-80

(5) Pienta KJ, Naik H, Akhtah A, et al. "Inhibition of spontaneous metastasis in a rat prostate cancer model by oral administration of modified citrus pectin." J Natl Cancer Inst 1995; 87: 348-353

(6) Strum S, Scholz M, McDermed J, et al. "Modified citrus pectin slows PSA doubling time: A pilot clinical trial. Presentation," International Conference on Diet and Prevention of Cancer, Tampere, Finland. May 28, 1999 - June 2, 1999.

(7) Glinsky VV, Huflejt ME, Glinsky GV, et al. "Effects of Thomsen-Friedenreich antigen-specific peptide P-30 on beta-galactoside-mediated homotypic aggregation and adhesion to the endothelium of MDA-MB-435 human breast carcinoma cells." Cancer Res

2000; 60: 2,584-8.

(8) Naik H, Pilat MJ, Donat T, et al. "Inhibition of in vitro tumor cell-endothelial adhesion by modified citrus pectin: a pH modified natural complex carbohydrate." Proc Am Assoc Cancer Res 1995: 36: Abstract 377

(9) Platt D, Raz A. "Modulation of the lung cell colonization of B16-F1 melanoma cells by citrus pectin." J Natl Cancer Inst 1992; 18: 438-42

(10) http://www.cancer.org/docroot/ETO/content/ ETO_5_3X_Modified_Citrus_Pectin.asp

Giving Patients a Shot at a Cancer-Free Future

(1) International Journal Cancer 2008; 122(2): 461-7